Digestive
By Dr. D. M.

*The following lectures on Digestive 1
Borland at the London Homœopathic H*

In approaching the subject, Dr. Borland took the drugs possessing a definite affinity for the digestive tract in their symptomatology, and picked out the outstanding distinguishing points between them. The notes contain much valuable detail born of personal experience, and manifest a wide knowledge of the subject.

AESCULUS

FROM the digestive angle, *Aesculus* is indicated usually in the rather older patient, the oldish man, who is beginning to break down a little. He is always rather heavy and dull, and there is a good deal of generous venous congestion, slightly congested veins, very often slightly dilated capillaries which are very obvious, and the patient is dull, heavy, and rather depressed. In most instances you will get a history that the patient has been quite a good liver; he has done himself pretty well and his digestion is beginning to give out.

The *Aesculus* patient usually complains a good deal of heartburn, with troublesome acid eructation. And the eructation is fairly typical; it is a very nasty, bitter, greasy type of eructation. He also tells you that very often after a decent meal, with that eructation he begins to gulp up little mouthfuls of sourish food.

Then, always you will get a complaint of fullness and discomfort immediately after a meal, sometimes amounting to actual pain, usually of a burning character, and this discomfort often continues right along to the second meal, which for a time gives him some relief.

On occasion you will get the story of this fullness and eructation going on to actual vomiting, the patient gulping up small quantities, mouthfuls, of food, which are sour or bitter, and of his going on doing this till his stomach is empty, when he feels very much more comfortable.

The next thing about this *Aesculus* patient is that with this general venous state, and with the general feeling of fullness in the abdomen, on examination you will always find a certain amount of hepatic enlargement. Associated with this, they often complain of backache, an aching pain in the back with a good deal of stiffness, and particularly they complain of difficulty in getting up out of a chair.

You have seen the congested old man in the club very often, a typical picture sitting back in an easy chair, and you have seen him struggling up out of his chair and holding his back—that is typical of *Aesculus*.

As a rule, the appetite is not good. They complain of a general lack of appetite, but usually, there is considerable thirst. These patients always suffer from constipation, and they are liable to get attacks of very painful hæmorrhoids, a feeling as if the rectum were full of sharp little sticks; and extreme pain on attempting to defecate.

They are always sensitive to pressure on the abdomen, or to tight clothing, and they always feel at their worst in the mornings when they wake. If they have an after-lunch nap, they wake feeling more bloated, more congested, and they have more eructation. They are also always sensitive to hot, stuffy atmospheres.

It is most important to get a knowledge of your drug as a whole and not to prescribe on a few well-known characteristics. For instance, the *Lachesis* patient has very much the same sort of temperature reactions as the *Aesculus* patient, very much the same venous congestion, very much the same distension, and also the marked aggravation after sleep; and yet mentally the two are poles apart.

Aesculus patients have the dull lethargy of the venous patient, who is just heavy, and sluggish, and wants to sit back in his chair; while *Lachesis* has all the mental activity, acute loquacity, and suspicion which immediately make you realise that you are dealing with a different type altogether.

Aesculus is the picture one tends to associate with the man who has done himself very well all his life; he is getting on in years, towards the seventies, and is beginning to go to pieces. Very often you will get a history that, during latter years, he has had very troublesome rheumatic pains, which tend to wander about from one place to another, and they are pretty sharp in character.

He is the type of patient who normally gets a dose of *Sulphur* from most of us, and we are rather worried and disappointed because he does not respond as a *Sulphur* patient should do. It is not really the patient's fault: it is ours.

ANACARDIUM

IT is well known that *Anacardium* is one of the routine medicines for pyloric or duodenal ulcers. But, unfortunately, from the homœopathic standpoint, the knowledge does not help much in being sure when to give it, and, merely for the local condition, it is most disappointing.

It is one of the fascinations, but one of the trials, of homœopathy, that one case of duodenal ulcer responds to *Anacardium* but the next one does not—it is one of the things that keeps up one's interest in the work. One can get a fairly definite picture of the *Anacardium* make-up, and link it on to the typical diagnostic symptoms of pyloric or duodenal ulcer.

The first thing about *Anacardium* patients is that they are always intensely irritable, bad-tempered, liable to curse and swear; but, and this is a diagnostic point for *Anacardium*, they are cowardly. If anyone stands up to their cursing, they simply crumple up, and have got no stuffing at all. It is obvious and very different from the *Nux* and *Hepar* make-up.

The next thing about them is that they suffer from an extreme feeling of indecision. They worry about things, they cannot make up their minds, and this worry and nervous fret is liable to bring on an attack of pain. Another point is that any excitement is also liable to produce an attack of abdominal pain.

Then, again from the prescribing point of view, it is helpful to remember that most of these *Anacardium* patients have a blunting of all their senses. Their sense of hearing is blunted. Their sense of smell is either blunted or disturbed. It is sometimes very acute for particular smells, and they sometimes have a nasty odour in the nose, but often the sense of smell is blunted.

The next thing that is a help in your drug selection is that these patients are rather insensitive to their surroundings. They do not fuss about things, untidiness does not worry them in any way. This is important because so many of the other drugs run exactly the opposite way.

Another symptom of which *Anacardium* patients complain is that they are liable to get sudden attacks of very profuse salivation. And not infrequently these patients have a rather offensive odour from the breath.

Usually they are moderately thirsty. But any cold food or drink—cold drink particularly—is liable to bring on an attack of acute pain. Another point is that *Anacardium* patients are all particularly aggravated by soup, which is liable to produce a very acute heartburn.

Anacardium patients often complain of a feeling of nausea in the morning on getting up. They often get a return of this when they begin to get hungry, and it is usually relieved by food. They also complain of a good deal of gurgling in the abdomen, rather than of actual distension. They have a sensation of a hard plug pressed into the epigastrium; this becomes steadily more acute, then they get a gurgle and the pain begins to subside.

As a rule, while these patients are eating they are fairly comfortable, and their comfort may last anything up to a couple of hours after a meal; then the pain begins to return. And it is usually a blunt pain.

Anacardium patients are always chilly. They are very sensitive to a cold draught; not at all keen on being out of doors, and yet there is one oddity about them—they get an astonishing amount of relief from exposure to the heat of the sun.

These patients always get a rather urgent call to stool; very often an urgent desire with inability to expel the stool, or else a good deal of difficulty and yet the stool is quite soft. In appearance, the typical *Anacardium* stool is pale, colourless, almost bileless. But not infrequently *Anacardium* patients have typical tarry stools, associated with a leaking ulcer.

The local abdominal pain is usually better for warm food, although any kind of food will relieve it with the exception of cold things. Not every duodenal ulcer calls for *Anacardium*, and it is only when you get the additional *Anacardium* symptoms that *Anacardium* will do good.

ARGENTUM NITRICUM

THE condition I tend to associate with *Argentum nit.* is the typical flatulent dyspepsia. It is indicated in definite gastric ulcer, but always a gastric ulcer which is associated with intense flatulence; a feeling of acute distension and other *Argentum nit.* symptoms referred to later.

The picture is of a nervous make-up—the typical anticipation neurosis which one commonly associates with *Argentum nit.* in all its complaints. Not infrequently this remedy is indicated in people who have been overworking, getting overtired, and whose digestion is giving out in consequence.

And these patients as a rule give the history that the first sign they get of becoming overtired is a sense of brain fag and the development of headache, coming on usually at the end of a day's work. And with that brain fag they get the feeling that they will not be able to carry on with their work, that they are going to have a nervous breakdown, or that they are going to have a gastric or duodenal ulcer.

They always have a marked sensitiveness to heat in any form, particularly close rooms, a stuffy atmosphere of any kind; and when they feel below par they develop an acute sensitiveness to any crowded place; a roomful of people; a theatre; a church; in fact a crowd of people anywhere.

All their digestive upsets are liable to be brought on, or made very much worse, from anticipating any important engagement which they have to keep. One of their most troublesome complaints is a feeling of intense abdominal distension, with violent efforts to bring up wind which they cannot expel, and then, after the effort has stopped, the wind gurgles up on its own account.

Very often you will hear the statement that when the pain is very acute, and they feel they are full to bursting point, they get marked relief from very dilute alcohol. It seems to break the wind, and they immediately become very much more comfortable.

In acute digestive upsets they develop an extreme desire for cold foods, cold drinks, iced foods, and as they have a definite desire for sweet things in any form, you find the *Argentum nit.* patients have a strong desire for ice cream. The cold foods and cold drinks seem to relieve the abdominal pain, but, as a rule, ice cream makes them worse.

They are very fond of sweets which always tend to increase their digestive difficulty. The appetite is usually fairly good, and these patients have a marked desire for strong-tasting, pungent food.

Very often there is a history of the pains developing immediately after the patient has taken any food. They continue getting worse for about an hour, and then there is vomiting, with relief. Sometimes the pain does not develop until about half an hour after a meal, and then becomes steadily worse until the patient vomits.

The pain usually starts right in the middle of the epigastrium and tends to spread from there round towards the left side of the abdomen under the left ribs. In acute gastritis or gastric ulceration, they get a good deal of vomiting, and the vomit may be blood-streaked or definite coffee-grounds.

These patients often suffer from quite acute nausea, and occasionally you come across an *Argentum nit.* patient who tells you that a sour drink will relieve the nausea, but usually the *Argentum nit.* gastric upsets are made much worse by sour fluids or sour food.

There is frequently a history of a chronic, very troublesome diarrhœa. Associated with that, there is a very useful point to remember as regards the appearance of the tongue.

When the disturbance is mainly of the upper digestive tract, the typical *Argentum nit.* tongue is a rather pale, flabby tongue, which is somewhat dry. But where there is much chronic bowel irritation, the tongue is liable to become smoother, redder, and looks rather as if the papillæ had been flattened out. It is still dry, and the mouth is still hot, but the appearance is quite different from that in the acute gastric upsets.

ARSENICUM ALBUM

THERE are indications for *Arsenicum alb.* in a variety of pathological conditions; in an acute gastritis, an acute gastro-enteritis, a gastric ulcer, or a gastric carcinoma. But no matter what the pathological condition is, unless you get the other *Arsenicum* indications the drug is not going to help. For instance, an acute gastro-enteritis, with vomiting and diarrhœa, as the result of food poisoning, may call for *Arsenicum.*

Not all such cases, however, call for it, and unless the other indications are present, *Arsenicum* will not do any good. For instance, one essential symptom in these *Arsenicum* cases is an intense burning pain, whether the lesion be in the stomach or the bowel. These burning pains are relieved by either external heat applied to the abdomen, or by taking mildly warm fluids; and definitely aggravated by cold.

In general make-up the *Arsenicum* patient is always extremely distressed, very anxious, very worried and very much afraid. Always restless, always thirsty, and craves cold drinks as the mouth is burning hot. Any vomit is again burning hot, and scalds the throat. But if the patient takes a cold drink, it will increase the abdominal pain. The patient himself is always chilly.

There are one or two points which are useful to remember. In an *Arsenicum* gastritis, the patient will complain of intense burning pain in the stomach, may vomit up a little fluid or may vomit up a quantity of fluid, and the fluid may be anything from mucus to bile or blood, but it is always associated with the same burning character of pain, and the same extreme sensitiveness of the stomach to pressure.

When treating a case of that type, there is one thing to remember: the *Arsenicum* gastritis is particularly aggravated by milk. So never put that patient on to a milk diet. The best plan with your *Arsenicum* cases is to put them on to water, nothing else, for forty-eight hours. Although they do not like sweet things, and they rather jib at glucose, they stand it quite well.

There is an odd thing in this connection. In children one occasionally sees an *Arsenicum* gastritis in which the patient seems to be singularly tolerant of sweetened, condensed milk, although they cannot tolerate ordinary milk. I cannot explain why this is so, but in practice it is the case.

Owing to its periodicity *Arsenicum* is often helpful in treating recurring bilious attacks.

Arsenicum patients with gastro-intestinal upsets feel so awful, so ill, and they are so afraid, that they get a definite craving for stimulants of all kinds—alcohol, coffee, tea, anything that may stimulate them—and all stimulants aggravate their pains. Mostly they have an aversion to food of any kind, and a particular loathing of anything fatty or greasy.

In *Arsenicum* cases the stools are very varied—acute watery diarrhœa with just little flecks of mucus in it, acute bile-laden stools, absolutely clay-coloured stools associated with an acute hepatitis, or a tarry stool associated with a gastric ulcer or a gastric carcinoma.

AURUM METALLICUM

INDICATIONS for *Aurum* occur in the typical malignant stomach. There are one or two very definite indications which point to such a case. *Aurum* is indicated for the patient who has realised that he is up against a malignancy, or at least a very serious illness, and he is very hopeless about the outcome of it.

The patient is singularly obstinate and does not always carry out instructions; he gets an idea into his head, either that it is no good his doing anything, or that something of which he has heard or read is going to cure him, and it is very difficult to persuade him otherwise.

As far as the appearance of the patient goes, many of these *Aurum* patients have, or have had, a definite cardiac lesion of some kind and are quite liable to have a good deal of colour, very often the sort of mitral flush associated with the cardiac lesion. Add to that the symptom that all these *Aurum* patients have a definite desire for air; they want plenty of fresh air circulating about them.

They get flushed and hot and when they are feeling particularly depressed, heavy and miserable, are very often helped for the time being by bathing, or by sponging the face and neck, in cold water.

The next thing is that most of these *Aurum* patients have a good appetite, very often an inordinate appetite, but it is not so much gastric symptoms which are relieved by eating or aggravated by hunger as the patient's general feeling. He feels very much better in himself after a meal, and he is very much worse if he is hungry—more depressed, more miserable, more disheartened.

In addition, these patients get a definite hunger pain which is relieved very often by eating, but they are much more likely to get a feeling of intense fullness, pressure, and weight in the upper part of the abdomen. Very often that feeling of fullness is more marked, or more complained of, in the left part of the upper abdomen than the right, although the majority of these cases have definite hepatic enlargement.

This may be the general enlargement due to cardiac back-pressure, the ordinary smooth, hard, congested liver, or it may be an irregular enlargement due to secondaries in the liver.

One peculiar symptom comes in here. The patient is rather hot-blooded, and yet with this feeling of drag and heaviness in the abdomen he very often complains that when it is bad he suffers from intensely cold legs and feet, very often they are icy cold, which is in contrast to the general hot-blooded state. And, not infrequently in these carcinomata where *Aurum* is indicated, there is quite early development of ascites.

As regards their appetite, they usually develop a definite craving for alcohol, coffee, very often for milk, and have a marked aversion to meat. And very often there is a history of alternating attacks of diarrhœa and constipation.

BROMIUM

THE type of case with indications for *Bromium* is that where there is suspicious ulceration in the stomach, usually with a history of pain coming on immediately after food, and very often of definite coffee-ground vomit. As a rule, these gastric pains are worse during the latter part of the day, and worse at night, and there are various gastric, or appetite, symptoms which are helpful in the selection of *Bromium* for these patients.

For instance, they often have an acute desire for acids, although their pain, or discomfort, is markedly aggravated from taking acid foods; and the taking of acids will not infrequently produce a sudden violent diarrhœa, or an acute gastric irritation which sets up a very irritating cough.

In other words, the stomach cough of our infancy does exist, and you meet it in these *Bromium* patients. They also have as marked an intolerance to oysters as you associate with *Lycopodium*.

Another point that sometimes helps to a *Bromium* diagnosis is that these patients have an undue susceptibility to tobacco. It is the common practice, when treating gastric or duodenal ulcers, to forbid tobacco, and in *Bromium* cases it is an absolute necessity, because they are extremely sensitive to it. They often say that smoking will produce gastric pain almost immediately; even sitting in a room where people are smoking is often enough to upset them.

They also get a marked aggravation from hot foods or hot drinks. These increase the discomfort or pain, make them feel sick, and may actually make them vomit; and yet they have a strong dislike for cold things. They get a sensation of hunger—an empty feeling in their stomachs—which is relieved by taking food, although their actual pain is aggravated. So you very often get an apparent contradiction.

So far as the general make-up is concerned, there are one or two points which help in *Bromium* selection. The patients are definitely hot-blodded. They are sensitive to heat, to hot rooms, to stuffy atmospheres, but they are even more sensitive to draughts, particularly a draught of cold air. If they exert themselves, they often suffer from distressing palpitation. They are usually somewhat emaciated, and not infrequently you have a history of recurring sore throats, and often their tonsillar glands will still be somewhat enlarged.

Bromium patients are always depressed, and have a strange kind of indifference. The one thing the *Bromium* patient does not want to do is work of any kind; he simply has no interest in it, and he shies from it.

Although *Bromium* patients have a tendency to flush when they get hot, or when they are in a hot atmosphere, as a rule they are pale, rather an earthy colour; and they may be completely ashen in appearance if they have had much hæmorrhage. And with their coffee-ground vomits they very often have a fairly sluggish, long-standing ulcer, and a history of repeated tarry stools.

Finally, these *Bromium* patients often complain of a very salt taste in the mouth, particularly in the morning on waking.

CARBO VEGETABILIS

CARBO VEGETABILIS, is the drug everyone thinks of who has a patient suffering from flatulence. But, unfortunately, not all flatulent patients respond to *Carbo veg.*, and it is a help to have a fairly clear idea of the kind of flatulent patient who requires this drug and thrives on it astonishingly well.

Carbo veg. patients are of course flatulent, and the typical *Carbo veg.* patient is the atonic dyspeptic. As a rule, they give a history of chronic minor indigestion lasting over a long period. There are two classes of patients who give that history.

Firstly, the thin, tall, atonic long-stomached patients whom one looks on as abdominal neurasthenics. They always have a feeling of abdominal discomfort, and a feeling as if their clothes were too tight. These patients are always tired, always miserable and look unhealthy.

They are pale and sallow. To stimulate their appetites, they want something either very salty or very sweet; they have a craving for coffee, acid drinks or acid fruits. They usually dislike meat, and any fatty food. If you attempt to put them on to a milk diet, they dislike it and feel much worse on it; and it appears to give them a marked increase of flatulence.

The other type of *Carbo veg.* patients do not look abdominal neurasthenics at all. They are rather over-weight, look well-nourished, and give a history of over-eating and, probably, over-drinking for years, particularly taking very rich, indigestible food; and their digestion is beginning to fail.

They have the same feeling of distension and fullness in the abdomen as the first type, and they also have a lot of flatulence; but these overfed patients very often have much more burning discomfort than the emaciated ones. They are very liable to attacks of general abdominal colic or of definite hepatic colic, and very often have gallstones.

On account of having done themselves too well, these patients go off meat food, particularly rich, very fatty foods, because they are made uncomfortable by anything of that sort. They develop much the same group of symptoms as the abdominal neurasthenics—in other words, the craving for coffee and sour things, and they get the same discomfort afterwards; they are just blown out.

Both of these types find a certain amount of temporary relief from eructation, from getting rid of some of this flatulent distension.

That is the chronic state of *Carbo veg.* patients. But they also suffer from acute attacks in which they get definite burning, epigastric pain, which usually come on some little time after food. With these burning pains, they very soon develop definite colicky attacks, which tend to recur, and which become more and more troublesome for about a couple of hours after eating.

At the end of that time they usually bring up a quantity of wind and the attack subsides for the time being. Instead of bringing up wind, they may have a sudden gurgle in the abdomen and the whole trouble subsides.

If these patients take anything in the way of ice cream, very iced water, or iced wine, it is liable to produce an almost immediate feeling of distension and acute abdominal colic. They go out and have a large dinner, take a quantity of slightly sour iced wine with it, and get acute abdominal distension. Add to that the little excitement of an after-dinner speech, and these patients collapse with acute heart failure.

The overfed type of *Carbo veg.* patients normally suffer from a somewhat torpid liver, which is usually a little enlarged, and they almost always suffer from constipation. The neurasthenic type also suffer from constipation, but they do not usually get the enlargement of the liver, although it may be palpable on account of the general visceroptosis.

There is one other complaint which both types of *Carbo veg.* patients frequently make. During their abdominal discomfort, when they are just feeling a bit distended and raw inside, they get a sudden flow of saliva into the mouth, and very often it is so extreme that it suddenly runs out of the mouth. This happens more during the night than during the day; they wake up and find their mouth full of saliva, and it may trickle out on to the pillow.

All these *Carbo veg.* patients, whatever their type, are sensitive to cold, are rather chilly, suffer from cold hands and feet, and yet all have a definite air-hunger. They are uncomfortable in an airless atmoshphere and, like the *Pulsatilla* patients, often feel definitely cold in a stuffy atmosphere.

As regards potency, I find that the over-fed type of *Carbo veg.* does well on a single dose of a high potency. In the case of the abdominal neurasthenic, however, you are better to give low rather than high potency, and I should start off with a 30.

Although *Carbo veg.* is usually indicated for an **atonic stomach** rather than for an **ulcer**, there are occasionally indications for it in chronic ulcer where there is delay at the pylorus and a dilated stomach as a result. Strangely enough, you sometimes get indications for *Carbo veg.* in ulceration at the cardiac end of the stomach, or the lower end of the œsophagus, and you quite frequently get indications for *Carbo veg.* in œsophageal carcinomas.

After patients with œsophageal carcinoma have swallowed their food, they get exactly the same feeling; they are filled up almost to bursting point; and then there is either eructation with a little fluid and relief, or there is a gurgle and the fluid goes through, giving relief. Patients have come into hospital unable to pass anything—or, possibly, only a little fluid—through the stricture, and on *Carbo veg.* have gone out after a few months, on a solid or semi-solid diet.

I usually start these œsophageal carcinomas on a low potency. Up to the present I have given them 30, though I should probably go lower still and give 12. A dose once a day for three, four or five days, and then stop the administration and watch the effect.

Whenever there are signs of increased difficulty, start the administration again, giving a dose every day for another four or five days and then stop again. In most cases the appetite has steadily increased each time the drug was repeated. Each time I repeat the drug I change the potency. I start off with 30, go on to 200 when I have to repeat; next time 1m, then 10m. I have not seen any cases where I have had to go higher than 10m.

I started to change the potency in this way because, in his last pronouncement on the question of potency, Hahnemann seemed to hint that if you changed it you could repeat more quickly than you could if you kept to the original one. It has been tried out in this country, and it is confirmed by experience. If you repeat the drug in the same potency you have to wait longer than if you give it in a different potency.

It does not seem to matter whether you increase or decrease the potency so long as you alter it. For instance, if you have given 200, it does not seem to matter whether you go up to 1m or down to 30; the important point is that you must alter the potency.

CAUSTICUM

CAUSTICUM is one of the most useful drugs we have for a type of patient that is very difficult to handle. For the rather broken down, chronic dyspeptic. Broken down in health, rather shaky, very depressed, very hopeless and very miserable. They give you a history of chronic indigestion, and what makes you think of *Causticum* is that, whenever the wind changes into a cold, dry quarter they are certain to get an attack of indigestion.

Another indication for *Causticum* is that these patients are very liable to develop a stiff neck, stiff back, stiff arm or a stiff muscle somewhere, from exposure to the same kind of cold, dry wind.

They suffer a great deal of abdominal discomfort. They describe their complaints in a variety of ways—a burning sensation in the stomach, a feeling that it is constantly out of order, a constantly soured stomach, a feeling as if everything fermented when it was swallowed—just the hundred and one expressions that you get from the chronic dyspeptic.

The symptom that indicates *Causticum* is that in spite of this spoiled stomach, they are painfully hungry all the time, though they cannot bear the thought of eating. If they want anything at all, they want something with a definite taste about it; pungent food of some kind, smoked meats, acid beer. They have a definite aversion to sweet foods, pastries, cakes, delicacies of most kinds.

Another interesting thing which always points to *Causticum* is that after a meal they are very liable to develop acute thirst with a desire for cold drinks—and yet, if they take very cold drinks after a meal, they get acute abdominal pain.

In their gastric attacks, *Causticum* patients get a certain amount of eructation or, more frequently, a feeling of sour fluid coming up into the throat. They may actually vomit, in which case the vomit is very sour and seems to scald the throat. After any starchy food they are liable to become flatulent, distended and very uncomfortable. And they usually suffer from pretty obstinate constipation.

As far as their actual lesion is concerned, I think chronic gastritis is the most common, but there are also indications for *Causticum* in cases of definite gastric ulcer.

CHELIDONIUM

CHELIDONIUM is one of the most satisfactory medicines because its indications are so clear. It is mainly indicated in cases of gastric catarrh, either acute or chronic, gastro-duodenal catarrh or catarrhal conditions of the gall bladder.

The textbooks say that *Chelidonium* patients are very heavy and lethargic, but I have seen quite a number of *Chelidonium* patients who were neither heavy nor lethargic. They have a certain amount of difficulty in concentration, and a good deal of forgetfulness; they are very often depressed, and are liable to have a good deal of anxiety; but normally I have not found the dull lethargy which is described in the textbooks.

Very often there is much restlessness, and the patients will complain of a strange and very distressing abdominal sensation, which is so acute that it makes them feel they will go crazy. They dislike any mental effort, and they dislike having to talk—I have noticed this very strikingly in quite a number of *Chelidonium* cases.

The patients as a whole are sensitive to heat, they are warm-blooded. This is worth remembering because their local gastric digestive symptoms are aggravated by anything cold and relieved by heat, although the patients themselves are aggravated by heat.

The tongue in *Chelidonium* cases is sometimes helpful. Many cases have a peculiarly pointed, narrow tongue, very often with a yellowish coat. And one surprising thing is that in spite of the tongue being narrow, it shows the imprint of the teeth at the sides.

Mostly, the patients complain of a very unpleasant, bitter taste—although sometimes it is just a horrible, spoiled taste—associated with the collection of a good deal of tough mucus in the mouth. With the complaint of a bitter taste, they are liable also to have attacks of sudden acute salivation.

The discomfort of which these patients complain is distinctive. They feel as if they had something tight round the upper part of the abdomen, almost like a band or a string. That is a constant sensation. It varies a little and sometimes goes on to a feeling of general abdominal fullness, particularly—again—in the upper part of the abdomen and more marked on the the right side.

With the general feeling of distension, is the complaint of acute, shooting pains which stab through from the front and usually go through to the back in the region of the right scapula. These sudden shooting pains are quite frequently accompanied by a colicky sensation and are not infrequently followed by an attack of pretty profuse vomiting, the vomit consisting of anything from glairy mucus to bile-stained material. It is unusual in *Chelidonium* to get much in the way of bleeding.

If there is much pain in the right half of the abdomen, it is usually aggravated by the patient's turning over on to the left side: it causes an increase of the feeling of distension and drag in the upper part of the abdomen. In the more acute colicky attacks, the pains are relieved by external warmth, aggravated by any abdominal pressure or by motion, and are made rather better by drawing up the legs and relieving the tension of the abdominal muscles.

Chelidonium patients have a good deal of flatulence, and they get great relief from bringing up wind. The striking characteristic of *Chelidonium* is the marked relief of pain from taking warm fluids—any warm, bland fluids, but particularly warm milk. Sometimes there is a craving for sour things, stimulants or beer, but any of these aggravate the pain.

They develop a marked aversion to meat, to fish in any form and to coffee. They always have a definite susceptibility to tobacco; smoking will bring on an attack of acute distension in the abdomen and may produce an attack of acute pain. The patients feel hungry, and get a certain amount of relief immediately after eating, particularly if the food is warm.

There are two main types of *Chelidonium* cases. In one the gall bladder is infected, and the patient is definitely jaundiced, has a bileless stool and a bile-stained urine. The kind of case in which *Chelidonium* is helpful is the one in which the patient is having irregular rigors, with rises of temperature, acute gall bladder pain and a feeling of general heat and exhaustion. In these cases, the rigor is liable to occur about 3 o'clock in the afternoon.

There is a tendency for a second rigor to take place in the early hours of the morning, usually about 4 o'clock. So far as the more chronic catarrhal condition is concerned—gastric catarrh and gastro-duodenal catarrh—the maximum discomfort is liable to occur in the latter part of the afternoon from about 4 o'clock to 9 o'clock.

Contrasting with that first acute infective case, there is another type of *Chelidonium* case, in which there does not seem to be the same degree of infectivity, but in which you appear to get more organic disturbance, sometimes running to a definite carcinoma, associated with a much more earthy appearance of the skin, very often with a slightly jaundiced tinge in the eyes, definitely dark stools and urine that is free from bile. That type, when associated with the *Chelidonium* food modalities, responds very well indeed to *Chelidonium*.

Apart from the occurrence of bileless stools in *Chelidonium*, there is not infrequently a history of alternating attacks of constipation and diarrhœa. Quite often digestive attacks of this type are associated with sudden changes of the weather; if the weather suddenly becomes too hot or too cold, the *Chelidonium* patient is liable to have an upset.

There is one other point which is sometimes a help in a *Chelidonium* diagnosis. Associated with the gall-bladder or liver upsets, the *Chelidonium* patient is very liable to develop severe, troublesome neuralgia of the right side of the head and face, particularly spreading down behind the right ear. I have never been able to explain the neuralgia, but I have come across it several times without any local focus.

Chelidonium does not appear to have any definite solvent effect on gallstones themselves. It does diminish the congestion of the common duct and, if the stones are of manageable size, they are passed. I myself have never seen them dissolved under the administration of *Chelidonium*.

CHINA

CHINA is one of our most neglected digestive medicines. Formerly, it was used extensively but, for some reason, it has fallen into disuse in this country. One hardly ever sees it prescribed, which is a great pity. It would seem that this is because we have all come to look on *China* as a medicine which is prescribed merely for the result of loss of fluid or prolonged illness; we look on it as a general pick-me-up instead of considering it on its merits and prescribing it for the conditions which it fits. And there are some very definite indications for *China* in digestive disturbances.

The condition in which you will require it is the atonic dyspepsia, associated with a good deal of intestinal disturbance, probably amounting to a definite colitis. It is also indicated in chronic dyspepsias associated with definite hepatic disturbances, which may go on to the formation of actual gallstones. No matter what the type of lesion from which they are suffering, these patients always have the most intense flatulence.

They seem to manufacture gas, and the outstanding characteristic is that they seem to be able to bring it up in any amount. Watching these cases, it is clear that many of them are air swallowers, and it is not really a fermentation. They are so constantly uncomfortable that they are swallowing air all the time and blowing themselves out. They bring up a great deal, start swallowing again, and again blow themselves out.

Mentally, *China* patients are interesting. They are always depressed, very discouraged and they have a horrible sense of frustration. Very often you get the history of a severe illness as the onset of the trouble, as the result of which they become irritable and develop a general hyperæsthesia. They are sensitive to everything—noise, touch, odours of any kind, and very often develop a peculiar hyperæsthesia to taste. This is rather interesting because, in spite of their extremely acute sense of taste, quite a number of *China* patients develop a craving for all sorts of highly tasting food—pungent, spicy things—in order to tickle their appetites.

All *China* patients are intensely chilly, very sensitive to cold draughts and want to be warmly covered up all the time. To this symptom of general chilliness you can add a *China* peculiarity: the patients complain of intense coldness in the stomach.

The tongue in the typical *China* case tends to be flabby, toneless and rather pale in colour; and they complain of an intensely bitter or salty taste. Not infrequently you meet a patient who complains of a horrible, slimy feeling in the mouth and, when that is present, they usually develop an intense antipathy to butter or greasy food of any kind.

There are various disturbances of the appetite. Some *China* patients have a horrible, gnawing, empty feeling and yet no real appetite for their food at all. They are quite indifferent about starting a meal, but their appetite seems to return once they begin. And they always get an increase of their flatulence and distension immediately after food. With that distension they begin to eructate, and this eructation may go on to definite vomiting, the vomit being of sour mucus which may be bile-stained or contain traces of blood.

Many of these patients eat quite well, taking a reasonable quantity of food, yet nearly all of them are emaciated. Not infrequently you come across a case in which the patient suffers from flatulent dyspepsia which is accompanied by the passage of undigested food in mucous stools. These cases give a definite history of night sweats and, in spite of a good appetite which is, in fact, frequently abnormally large, the patients are noticeably emaciated.

Associated with the digestive upsets in *China* patients, you will almost always get a complaint of intense weariness and a general aching pain all over. They say they feel just as if they had done a great deal of hard physical labour and were completely tired out.

In the attacks of acute abdominal pain, the abdomen becomes hyperæsthesic on the surface to light touch, and yet the pain is relieved by firm pressure. These chronic dyspeptics are very liable to suffer from attacks of facial or definite dental neuralgia; it seems to pick up the trigeminal nerve. These neuralgias, again, are very sensitive to any draught of cold air, very sensitive to light touch, definitely helped by firm, steady pressure, and relieved by warmth.

All *China* patients give a history of absolute intolerance to any acid—sour food or sour drink. These immediately produce a feeling of acute, abdominal discomfort, increased abdominal distension, general gurgling in the abdomen and an attack of diarrhœa.

In dealing with a *China* colitis, you will find that the patients complain that they are liable to get an attack of diarrhœa immediately after food. In addition, they get very troublesome nocturnal diarrhœa. The motion usually consists of a mucous stool with a quantity of undigested material, and is passed to the accompaniment of large quantities of flatus.

In the chronic *China* patient there tends to be a certain amount of enlargement of the liver, usually a hard liver; and there is sometimes a certain amount of enlargement of the spleen.

It has been said that in many cases of gallstones, associated with that type of flatulent dyspepsia, you can get immense relief—in fact, many homœopaths declare that you can get solution of the gallstones—by the continued administration of *China* 6 over a length of time.

In this connection it may be worthwhile to mention *Colocynth*. Where you have a hepatic colic which has responded to *Colocynth*, you will very often find that *China* is your most useful follow-up after the immediate gallstone colic is over.

If you just think about *Colocynth* for a moment, I am sure that you will realise that the abdominal picture is very similar to that of *China*. It is more a spasm of the circular fibres in *Colocynth*, and more a paralytic condition in *China*; with the result that in *China* there is flatulence, whereas in *Colocynth* there is irregular spasm and colic. In *China*, there is aggravation from sour foods; in *Colocynth*, very often, the colic is brought on by taking icy cold foods, but it may also be produced by sour things, particularly cold sour things.

The two drugs have almost the same modalities: they both have definite relief from pressure, definite amelioration from warmth and definite aggravation from cold. So it is not surprising that *China* should very often take up the work where *Colocynth* has relieved the acute spasm.

Incidentally, *Colocynth* has a facial neuralgia which is almost identical with that of *China*. The modalities are practically the same. The *Colocynth* neuralgia is not quite so sensitive to cold, though it has the same relief from firm pressure, and it has exactly the same distribution over the trigeminal nerve. It is, therefore, not surprising that these drugs run pretty closely together.

CONIUM

CONIUM is a very useful medicine in malignant conditions of the stomach—either chronic ulcers that have become malignant or, more commonly, malignant growths round about the pylorus, usually with secondary deposits in the liver.

Many of the patients who ought to have *Conium* are given one of the sodium salts instead, the reason being that they have a definite dislike of people, want to be left alone and quiet, and have a definite craving for salt. But there are distinct differences in the mentality of *Conium* and of sodium patients. *Conium* patients do not want to be disturbed, but they dislike being entirely alone. They are depressed, but it is a very quiet, gentle melancholy in *Conium*, not the acute mental depression of the sodium patients. And there is very often a strange superstitiousness in *Conium* which is not usually associated with sodium cases.

Naturally, where you are dealing with a thing like an abdominal carcinoma, the patient is weak, tired out, and any mental effort is a great strain. One thing that helps you to your diagnosis of *Conium* is that this weakness is accompanied by definite tremulousness. It is also accompanied by very marked vertigo, particularly on any sudden movement: the patient, who has been sitting quietly, suddenly gets up from his chair, and becomes giddy; or he turns suddenly in bed and immediately everything begins to swing round.

As regards the appetite, there may be hunger—sometimes almost a craving for food—or there may be complete loss of appetite. A point to remember is their definite craving for salt. And not infrequently there is a marked aversion from bread in any form.

There are one or two interesting points in connection with the stomach symptoms. In *Conium* you frequently get a history that on swallowing food the patient feels as if it is stuck in his throat. Well, you get much the same condition in *Natrum mur.*—the ordinary *Natrum mur.* spasm—but, in *Conium*, the patient feels as if something rose up from the stomach and blocked the food that was coming down: *Natrum mur.* cases feel as if the œsophagus closed on the food and prevented it passing further. Then, apart from eating, *Conium* patients are apt to get the same sort of sensation of something rising up into the throat, and it often produces a quite irritating cough.

These patients commonly complain of acute heartburn and violent, stabbing pains, feeling exactly as if a knife were sticking into the right side of the upper abdomen, passing across to the left side and producing intense nausea. They frequently vomit and the material is always very stringy in character and difficult to get up. It may consist of stringy mucus, bile or coffee-ground material.

Another complaint of *Conium* patients is that, some little time after eating, they get a feeling as if the contents of the stomach were being pushed out through a narrowed pylorus. They tell you that they can often feel a definite lump rising up about the pyloric area as the food attempts to force its way through. And where these patients are suffering from a pyloric carcinoma you can feel the tumour.

In these cases you get early involvement of the liver, which is enlarged and irregular. Often they complain of very sharp, tearing, stitching pains in the liver. Associated with the early dissemination into the liver there will almost certainly be enlarged abdominal glands as well, very often hard lumps in the abdomen, and the whole abdomen very sensitive.

The patient often complains that, apart from these hard lumps, there are areas in the abdomen which seem to come up in hard knots, as if there were intestinal spasm. But, rather than the spasmodic colic you associate with some of the other drugs, in these *Conium* patients you get acute cutting pains. Most of the gastric pains come on about a couple of hours after a meal, and they are all of this forcing character.

Many of these patients suffer from alternate attacks of diarrhœa and constipation. Whether they are constipated or have diarrhœa they are mostly very exhausted after the bowels have acted; they feel very shaky and almost faint.

With their abdominal carcinomas, these patients frequently have disturbances of the bladder, usually a partial paralysis in which the urine stops and starts and they have difficulty in completely emptying the bladder.

There is one other point which is sometimes a help. In addition to the cough which is associated with their gastric discomfort, *Conium* patients often complain bitterly of a very dry spot in the larynx, which they cannot moisten and which sets up a constant, irritating cough.

GRAPHITES

G RAPHITES is one of the routine medicines prescribed in cases of duodenal ulcer but, unless the definite *Graphites* indications are present, one does not obtain a satisfactory result and, as there are quite a number of other drugs which also have a bearing on duodenal ulcers, it is important to have the *Graphites* picture quite clear.

The majority of *Graphites* patients are rather overweight; they tend to be fat. They are usually pale in colour, although sometimes they have a fair amount of colour. One woman with a duodenal ulcer responded very well to *Graphites* and she had quite a high colour.

Mentally, they tend to be rather despondent, depressed and lacking in energy. It is not so much mental stamina they lack, but actual drive. They cannot make up their minds, are hesitant in all they do, and worry about their affairs. Quite frequently you are told that the actual acute attack for which they consult you was precipitated by a period of unusual mental stress.

As a rule, these patients are chilly and feel the cold a good deal. But they are very sensitive to any stuffy atmosphere or lack of air. If you enquire into their history carefully, you often find that they have suffered at some time from some degree of skin disturbance, usually an eczematous type of eruption—very often eczematous patches at the back of the ears. Or, they may have had digestive upsets with attacks of piles, very troublesome peri-anal fissures, and eczema.

As regards their actual complaints, they have a beastly, spoiled stomach which feels just out of order; they feel rather sick and get a good deal of eructation. That goes on to more acute attacks in which they have heartburn or actual acute pain, which is usually of a griping character and, when this is extreme, there may be attacks of vomiting.

Not infrequently these patients say that with the attack of pain and feeling of sickness there is a horrible, sudden sensation of extreme weakness—a feeling as if they were going to faint. Following this sensation of faintness, in quite a number of cases, there has been vomiting of blood or, short of that, definite melæna for the next day or two. So this feeling of collapse is apparently associated with a sudden gastric hæmorrhage.

In addition to the more or less chronic state, *Graphites* patients suffer from definite hunger pains which gradually develop about two hours after food, and are relieved by eating.

Considering actual likes and dislikes, one of the outstanding differentiating *Graphites* symptoms is the marked aversion to sweets. There is very often an aversion to salt also, but this is not so marked.

Frequently one comes across a patient who has a very definite aversion to animal food. This seems to be more mental than physical, for the patient will often say that the food tastes quite good if they can overcome the aversion, but they shy from taking animal food in any form.

With their acute attacks of heartburn, there is a feeling of intense heat in the stomach and throat and a desire for cold drinks, in order to cool down the stomach; but, as a rule, *Graphites* patients are aggravated by cold food. When they have pain they are relieved by warm drinks, very often especially relieved by warm milk.

These patients always complain of a good deal of abdominal flatulence, a feeling of general abdominal distension with indefinite griping pains. With these attacks of flatulence they feel a sudden rush of blood, a sudden flush of heat, to the face and head. With the general abdominal distension they are very intolerant of any tight clothing, it makes them more uncomfortable. And I have been told that, after one of the acute attacks, the patient developed a definite herpetic eruption round the abdomen.

Most *Graphites* patients are constipated, and their constipation is rather suggestive. They have periods when there is no inclination for the bowels to act; followed by a griping, colicky disturbance and then an action of the bowel in which they pass a very large stool accompanied by a quantity of white mucus. Normally, the stool tends to be palish but, after one of the acute attacks in which there is leakage from a gastric or duodenal ulcer, they have black, melæna stools.

Often *Graphites* patients complain of a very unpleasant taste in the mouth: either just a spoiled taste like the spoiled sensation they get in the stomach, or a bitter, salt taste. With this saltish, bitter taste they frequently develop little burning blisters on the side of the tongue.

There is one other point that sometimes helps in diagnosis: many of these *Graphites* patients develop a marked hyperæsthesia of the sense of smell, particularly to the odour of flowers. This is not constant, however, and others suffer from a chronic nasal catarrh in which the sense of smell is entirely lost; they have a yellowish, excoriating discharge, a tendency to develop cracks at the side of the nose, and small, slightly spreading eczematous patches.

As regards the actual pathological condition, most cases tend to develop a duodenal ulcer. In most of the satisfactory *Graphites* cases I have seen, actual ulceration has been demonstrated by a barium meal.

There is astonishingly little scarring after *Graphites*. I have found that the ulcer has disappeared and the duodenal cap returned practically to normal—as shown by X-ray examination—and it is quite insensitive to pressure. In any case, with persistent scarring I would give *Graphites* in low potency, say 6, for a week or two to see if it could be diminished.

HEPAR SULPHURIS CALCAREA

HEPAR SULPH. is another of the medicines which are neglected in digestive disturbances, and many cases in which we ought to give *Hepar sulph.* are given *Nux vomica* instead.

There are many similarities between these two medicines. Mentally they are very alike. They are both hyperæsthetic in every way; irritable, snappy, hasty in their movements, impatient and very chilly. In the majority of cases both *Hepar sulph.* and *Nux vom.* tend to be rather underweight, but usually *Hepar sulph.* patients have more colour; very often they have bright red cheeks instead of the sallow *Nux* appearance.

All the *Hepar sulph.* patients I have treated for digestive disturbances have had very unhealthy mouths; they have a tendency to caries of the teeth, unhealthy gums and very often a history of dental abscesses. Frequently the breath is offensive and there is an unpleasant—or definitely metallic—taste in the mouth.

Most *Hepar sulph.* patients tend to develop a horrible sensation of hunger in the middle of the morning—a very unpleasant, empty sensation. And with this they have an acute craving for highly seasoned, strong-tasting food of every kind.

One thing that always suggests *Hepar sulph.* is the fact that not only are the local gastric symptoms relieved by food, but the patients themselves feel a hundred per cent. better after a meal; it seems to lift them generally, quite apart from the relief of their local symptoms.

These patients usually suffer from a good deal of heartburn, with very troublesome, acid eructations.

Associated with the empty feeling in the stomach is a very distressing sensation of the whole abdominal contents hanging down; this is particularly increased by standing about or by walking. In spite of this sagging sensation, they are made uncomfortable by anything in the nature of abdominal support; external support of any kind seems to increase their distress. So, be a little careful of anything in the nature of a Curtis belt in the visceroptotic *Hepar sulph.* cases.

These patients are very liable to recurring attacks of vomiting—almost bilious attacks. The typical feature of the attack is that the patient feels horribly sick, makes violent efforts to vomit and, after severe retching, brings up a quantity of bile-stained fluid.

Associated with these bilious attacks the patient has acute, cutting pain, usually about the region of the umbilicus, accompanied by much rumbling in the abdomen and, sometimes, definite colic. With these general abdominal upsets troublesome attacks of acute diarrhœa are very liable to develop. The type of stool in *Hepar sulph.* cases is very offensive and fermenting. Often these people have had recurring attacks of this kind every spring and autumn for years, and while the attack lasts there is frequently profuse, sour-smelling, generalised sweat.

In addition to the craving for stimulating foods of all kinds, there is one *Hepar sulph.* characteristic which is sometimes a great help: with the digestive upsets there is very often a definite craving for vinegar. This is a clear *Hepar sulph.* pointer.

It is said that these patients have a marked craving for fat. I have not treated one who had a craving for fat during a digestive upset; but I have had quite a number of *Hepar sulph.* patients who had digestive upsets of this nature and who developed an acute aversion to anything greasy or fatty. So do not ignore this drug just because the patient does not have a craving for fat.

HYDRASTIS CANADENSIS

HYDRASTIS is one of the drugs required for the most serious types of abdominal trouble, usually a very acute gastritis, a gastric ulcer or a gastric carcinoma. The cases are always very serious, and the patients feel extremely ill. They are despondent rather than anxious about themselves, and very often feel so uncomfortable that they would be thankful to die. They are completely worn out and exhausted.

As a rule, they are pale and have rather a greasy appearance. Many of the *Hydrastis* patients I have seen have had very marked blackheads on the skin—a condition that one tends to associate with that kind of greasy complexion.

These patients complain of a horribly flat taste—nothing tastes good at all—and they very often complain of the tongue feeling as if it had been burned. The whole throat feels raw and sore, and they have the same rawness and soreness in the stomach.

As a rule, you are told that the patient vomits practically everything taken, except possibly a little milk and water. They complain of an acute burning pain and, associated with it, a feeling of emptiness. With this emptiness there is a complete loathing of food, and the sinking sensation seems to be worse if they take any food; it does not relieve them at all.

With this burning pain in the stomach, the patients very often have violent pulsation in the epigastrium, accompanied by acute palpitation.

All their distress is aggravated by taking bread, or any vegetables.

Very often in these cases there is an early development of jaundice, with a rather hard, somewhat tender liver. Owing to this torpid, heavy liver, there is often a dragging sensation and a good deal of burning pain in the hepatic region.

These patients have frequent attacks of colic—generalised colicky pains—in the abdomen, and they usually suffer from extreme constipation; it is almost impossible to get their bowels to act at all. Occasionally, however, one meets *Hydrastis* patients who have bouts of diarrhœa, in which they pass very bileless, almost colourless stools.

It is very similar to the picture described under *Arsenicum*, but without the *Arsenicum* distress, thirst, fear of death. In *Hydrastis* you have the despondent, dead-beat patient, instead of the anxious, thirsty *Arsenicum* patient.

IGNATIA AMARA

IGNATIA dyspepsias are rather common, and definite in their symptoms. Most of the *Ignatia* cases one meets are typical examples of nervous dyspepsias of various kinds; and they are always associated with the unexpectedness that you meet with in *Ignatia* in any condition.

For instance, in your *Ignatia* dyspeptic you will get a combination of complete lack of appetite with a craving for food; or there is a feeling of intense nausea associated with hunger—a horrible, empty, dragging feeling in the abdomen, with complete aversion to taking any food at all. These are typical of the contradictory conditions which one associates with *Ignatia* in any of its disturbances.

The most constant symptom running through all *Ignatia* digestive disturbances is that feeling of emptiness: most *Ignatia* patients seem always to be nibbling food of some kind. They very often tell one that they are so uncomfortable, particularly in the evening and night, that they simply must have some biscuits by their bed or they get no rest at all; and the same sort of thing applies throughout the day as well.

The next striking thing is that almost invariably their desires and aversions for food are very inconstant. For a week they may have a craving for one thing, then that craving entirely disappears and, for the next week, they may have just as marked an aversion to it.

Associated with that there is the complaint that the patient starts a meal quite hungry and interested and then, in the middle of the meal, all desire for food suddenly disappears—everything tastes unpleasant, flat, or insipid, and they want nothing more.

With their digestive disturbances, the majority of these patients have a certain amount of nausea, and very often there is a sudden regurgitation of food. This is usually rather bitter in taste, and may be associated with a good deal of flatulence and eructation, which comes on immediately after eating.

With that, you can link up the symptom that *Ignatia* patients suffer from very troublesome, persistent attacks of hiccough. These attacks are often very painful and difficult to control, but frequently you will find that they are relieved by taking something to eat.

One constant *Ignatia* symptom in their digestive disturbances is a complete intolerance of tobacco. The *Ignatia* patient is quite liable to feel sick, nauseated, or to get an acute attack of hiccough, if he smokes.

They suffer from a strange mixture of fullness and emptiness. Very often there is a feeling of extreme emptiness immediately after food, which is later followed by distension and fullness associated with a certain amount of shortness of breath and almost air-hunger or, even more frequently, a tendency to constant sighing.

Another symptom of which they often complain is definite colicky pains. And, again, the strange thing about these pains is that they are often relieved by eating.

The actual pathological condition from which *Ignatia* patients mostly suffer is simply a flatulent dyspepsia, without any definite organic lesion. In that state they develop an acute aversion to any warm food, and to meat; peculiarly, they are often more comfortable after taking some sour fluid or sour food.

But you cannot rely on these symptoms, because one week you may get them and the next week you may get entirely the reverse. One thing that is constant in the *Ignatia* patient, in addition to the intolerance of tobacco, is a marked intolerance of coffee. It increases their digestive disturbance, very often gives them a crampy pain, and may even set up definite hiccough and regurgitation of food.

All *Ignatia* patients suffer from troublesome, generalised abdominal flatulence. Often they have great difficulty in getting rid of it, and it is associated with very marked constipation. The constipation in *Ignatia* is much the type one associates with *Nux vomica*, that is to say, the constant, ineffectual urging to stool.

One is sometimes apt to confuse *Ignatia* with *Argentum nit.* which also has this intense abdominal flatulence. In both the flatulence is much aggravated by sweets, but the point to remember is that in *Ignatia* you get this flatulence associated with colic and constipation, whereas in *Argentum nit.* you get it associated with colic and diarrhœa.

Ignatia patients do get attacks of diarrhœa, but it is most commonly entirely painless, and is usually associated with some emotional disturbance—fright, shock or something similar—it is not usually the result of indiscretion in diet, nor is it the anticipation diarrhœa of *Argentum nit.*

In addition to their abdominal flatulence, *Ignatia* patients mostly complain of a horrible feeling of weakness in the abdomen, a dragging down sensation; and they all, in that weak state, are aggravated by any stimulants—alcohol, tea, coffee and, particularly, spirits in any form.

There are one or two small points about *Ignatia* which are sometimes suggestive. With their digestive upsets they tend to get a good deal of salivation, with a sourish taste in the mouth. Again, they complain very often of a troublesome tendency to bite the inside of the cheek.

On looking inside the mouth, you will find that the ampulla at the end of the parotid duct is very definitely swollen: it is in this region that the patient has this difficulty and tends to bite the slightly pouting mucous membrane on the inside of the cheek.

Ignatia patients, with all their flatulence, often develop an insatiable desire for bread, which is, needless to say, very inadvisable.

With their digestive upsets you find, of course, the ordinary unstable *Ignatia* make-up. These patients are excitable, or depressed and weeping; they want attention and sympathy, and yet they are very much more emotional if any sympathy is given to them. And frequently the commencement of their digestive history dates from some acute emotional upset, either emotional shock or nervous fright.

Ignatia is not a long-acting drug. In the typical *Ignatia* case I do not find that the action is much longer than three weeks, even in a very high potency.

IODIUM

IODIUM is one of the very interesting digestive drugs, and it covers a number of definite pathological conditions. There are three conditions which *Iodium* covers particularly well. The most important is chronic pancreatitis. The condition of second importance is a very chronic gastric carcinoma. The third is a cirrhotic liver, which may be a primary cirrhosis, a chronically inflamed liver or a liver with metastatic growths in it.

No matter what the pathological condition, there are certain constant factors which lead to the prescription of *Iodium*. My experience has been rather contrary to what is laid down in the textbooks of materia medica as to the *Iodium* make-up.

The textbooks all stress the intense irritability, the intense restlessness and the strung-up nervous state of *Iodium*. But in the cases in which I have seen *Iodium* helpful, a marked characteristic has been a general mild despondency.

The patients have always been rather mild, intensely scrupulous in all their dealings and somewhat timid. But it is that intense scrupulousness of the *Iodium* patient which, to my mind, is their outstanding characteristic.

As far as the irritability is concerned, in these digestive cases it is a symptom which tends to develop during the process of digestion, and is by no means a constant factor in the patient's make-up.

Another constant in *Iodium* patients is their tendency to become worried and anxious if their meal is delayed and they become at all hungry. They have a very marked desire for food. They do not necessarily want a great quantity at a time—in fact, they often are not able to eat much at all—but they have a very quickly recurring need for food and, if they do not get it, become worried, anxious, restless and distressed.

So far as their desire for food is concerned, they do not seem to have very definite cravings. Some have a marked desire for meat;

but, usually, it is food of any kind that the *Iodium* patient wants, more than any particular articles of diet.

These patients always have a good deal of generalised abdominal pain, the exact nature and situation depending to some extent on the pathological lesion. But in all these cases there is a certain amount of relief immediately after taking food.

In gastric carcinoma they often complain of a burning pain, associated with marked epigastric pulsation and quite extreme epigastric tenderness. In these gastric carcinomas the patients usually have rather a pale, yellowish complexion, with somewhat striking, bluish lips. This holds good for all the *Iodium* lesions, no matter what they are.

Both in gastric carcinomas and in pancreatic lesions, *Iodium* patients are liable to get attacks of acute salivation and vomiting, which are often extremely distressing. The tongue tends to be very dry, and patients often complain that it feels scalded or burned.

In spite of the general restlessness the patients often complain of extreme faintness on movement: sitting up, getting out of bed, standing, will bring this on—particularly when they are hungry.

In their gastric conditions they mostly suffer from obstinate constipation, which is a great trial to them, and is associated with marked abdominal distension. They may also get spasms of localised distension, which are extremely painful.

With that can be linked another *Iodium* symptom: the distension due to diffuse, generalised enlargement of the abdominal glands in carcinoma cases. You will get the same thing with the pancreatic lesions and, if you are dealing with a secondary hepatic carcinoma, you will find the enlarged glands there, too. The characteristic feature is that these glands are definitely tender on palpation, and they feel very, very hard.

As far as the pancreatic cases are concerned, *Iodium* patients suffer from the typical pancreatic pain, that is to say, a pain right across the upper part of the abdomen, about an inch above the umbilicus, associated with a horrible fullness, tenderness and an intense pressing feeling. Cases with these pancreatic lesions have attacks of diarrhœa, with very unpleasant, frothy stools.

Where you are dealing with the disturbances of the liver, whether as a primary cirrhosis or as a secondary carcinomatous condition, there is liable to be jaundice, but it is fluctuant in intensity; the jaundice is constant, but it varies in degree. These cases have clay-coloured stools, very often recurring attacks of exhausting diarrhœa, with somewhat frothy stools.

As regards results of treatment. In pancreatic cases, where there could be no question about the diagnosis, with definite fermentation of the stools, the patients have definitely improved after treatment. I have seen cases with definite masses of glands in the abdomen clearing up, and the patients' capacity for dealing with fats going up out of all recognition.

I do not say that these patients are cured. I have treated one or two of them who died. But their pain had been removed, their abdominal distension went down, they put on weight, they lost their hopeless outlook, and they lost their recurring attacks of diarrhœa. These patients do not get well, but it is astonishing what comfort you can give them.

I treat all carcinomas who have had X-rays with one of the radioactive salts as a first measure—to try to antidote the X-rays. Usually one of the radium salts, *Radium bromide* or *Radium iodide*. If there are any indications for *Iodium*, I prefer the *Radium iodide* to the *Radium bromide*.

Iodium is one of the very useful medicines for relieving those patients who normally go on to massive sedative treatment and have an appalling end. With the aid of *Iodium* it is astonishing what relief can be given to these patients, although it may not actually cure them.

In any of these cases I give the drug fairly frequently to begin with, and find it holds for longer and longer intervals; so I think there is no doubt that it definitely has a curative effect.

I have seen *Iodium* indicated in mammary carcinomas, but I have never had a clear indication for it in uterine carcinoma. I had a case once with a carcinoma of the tongue, and she did very well on *Iodium*. Eventually I lost sight of her and did not know the ultimate result. But the epithelioma of her tongue shrank to half the size, and the mass of glands in her neck almost disappeared.

KALIUM BICHROMICUM

THERE are three kinds of condition calling for *Kali bic*. First is the acute catarrhal condition of the mucous membranes of the digestive tract, acute gastritis, gastric catarrh, gastro-duodenal catarrh or gastro-enteritis. The catarrhal condition is much the commonest for which *Kali bic.* is indicated. Second is the definite ulcerative condition, particularly a gastric ulcer. And third is ulcerative colitis.

In all these cases you are dealing with a very typical patient. The *Kali bic.* patient tends to be fat, sluggish, restless, depressed and taciturn. You will usually get a history that these patients have been subject to chronic catarrh all their lives, and they mostly suffer from a degree of chronic nasal, or post-nasal, catarrh—very often with a perpetually choked sensation about the root of the nose.

All these patients suffer from wandering rheumatic pains. They are not very severe in character, but tend to wander about from one place to another, and are always relieved by motion.

Normally, the patients are rather pale, but with their digestive upsets they tend to become somewhat blotchy. Very often they suffer from acute attacks of acne.

Depending on the type of lesion, you find two kinds of tongue associated with *Kali bic.* In catarrhal conditions they tend to have a thickly coated tongue, particularly at the base, and they have a nasty, flat, bitterish or sweetish taste and a good deal of sticky saliva. The coating may be anything from sticky white to thick yellow, and the base is particularly affected.

In ulcerative conditions, especially in ulcerative colitis, you usually find a very dry, smooth, red, almost glazed tongue.

The commonest story given by these patients is that they have absolutely no appetite, and very often they have a loathing of food in the morning. It may be that they start their breakfast but about half-way through cannot continue with it. Or they may have the typical morning nausea, with complete inability to face breakfast at all.

After a meal they suffer from an intense feeling of fullness, heaviness and general malaise. This comes on quite soon after a meal, and is usually accompanied by a very unpleasant feeling of general chilliness. With this sensation of fullness, they are liable to have sudden attacks of nausea and vomiting.

The vomit in *Kali bic.* is very suggestive. It is sour in taste, contains a great amount of mucus, is difficult to expel, and the mucus hangs down from the patient's mouth.

There is one odd symptom of which these patients sometimes complain: a strange feeling of irritation in the throat. It feels as if they had a foreign body hanging on the soft palate, and intense nausea and even actual vomiting may be produced by it. Very often they describe it as the sensation of a hair on the back of the throat, or something of that nature. Not infrequently this is associated with their nasal catarrh and is, in fact, a string of mucus, which makes them retch and gag.

Kali bic. patients suffer from pretty extreme burning gastric pains, which may become very acute tearing pains going right through to the back between the scapulæ. When the pain is bad it is usually accompanied by a good deal of acute water brash.

During the day they mostly suffer from a general lack of appetite, and yet they feel faint and gone if they do not have some food. With this feeling of faintness there may be a suggestion of nausea, which is relieved by taking a little food.

These patients are usually thirsty and very often they develop a marked craving for beer and sour or bitter foods, all of which tend to aggravate their distress. In some of the ulcerative conditions, particularly if the ulcer is towards the pyloric end of the stomach, they suffer from definite hunger pains which come on about three hours after a meal.

A distinguishing point is that the pain goes on to actual vomiting, and the patients bring up typical stringy mucus, which may be actually blood-stained. And, with this ulcerative condition, *Kali bic.* patients are very liable to develop an extremely sore spot in a small area in the epigastrium.

There is one condition in which *Kali bic.* is almost specific: the gastritis associated with excessive beer drinking. It has the typical morning aversion to food, the typical glairy vomit associated with the beer drinker, the horrible slack inertia in the morning, the hunger and dislike of food, and the recurring attacks of nausea. *Kali bic.* will not only clear up the gastritis, but it will also stop the craving for beer.

In ulcerative colitis, *Kali bic.* patients have very acute, griping diarrhœic attacks. The diarrhœa is exceedingly suggestive: it is brown, frothy, watery, offensive and usually accompanied by the passage of a quantity of stringy mucus. Not infrequently there is a quantity of pus mixed up with the stool.

In the more chronic colitis cases, there is often a spring aggravation in *Kali bic.* patients. They are fairly comfortable during the rest of the year, but each spring the condition flares up again, and they get another bout of colicky griping and this violent, distressing diarrhœa.

Quite frequently, in *Kali bic.* digestive cases, there is a history that the patients have been subject to migraine attacks all their lives. These attacks are very typical. The patients have violent, sick headaches, associated with pain situated in one small spot above one eye. The pain gradually becomes more and more intense until it produces violent vomiting of typical, stringy mucus.

The particular point is that these migraine attacks are always associated with ocular disturbances—zigzags, disturbances of the field of vision, partial blindness, or something of that nature—preceding the onset of the acute pain.

One drug should be mentioned which does not come into these digestive drugs but which should always be remembered in association with these *Kali bic.* recurring migraine attacks characterised by disturbances of vision, pains in small spots and the typical stringy vomit—*Iris*. *Iris* has almost exactly the same symptom picture, and occasionally you will come across a patient you think is typical *Kali bic*, but whose migraines do not clear on it; and you will find it clears on *Iris*. The picture of the migraine attack is identical; it is impossible to distinguish one from the other. So, when you encounter an apparent *Kali bic.* migraine that does not respond, always remember *Iris*.

KALIUM CARBONICUM

KALI CARB. has a number of indications for digestive disturbances, varying from a general slacking down of digestion to typical flatulent dyspepsia and the development of gallstones; occasionally *Kali carb.* patients have very suggestive symptoms which point to an œsophageal obstruction, possibly an œsophageal spasm or sometimes a definite organic stricture.

But these symptoms alone do not help to select *Kali carb.* as the drug; you have to add them to the general picture which it is rather difficult to summarise. I give the one that has appeared as fairly typical, although it is not exactly what you find in the materia medica.

Kali carb. patients are usually somewhat anæmic, rather pale and always definitely chilly. They are sensitive people, dislike being alone, are rather worried—often particularly worried about their diseases and not a little frightened.

Mentally, their moods tend to alternate. At times they are quite cheery, at others they seem to be unduly depressed and liable to weep. Running through their make-up there is a strain of irritability. They are very easily irritated by noise, are often unduly sensitive to voices, and easily startled—any sudden touch or noise startles them.

Another fairly constant symptom is a tendency to a troublesome chronic nasal catarrh, usually associated with some crusting about the nostrils. With the chronic catarrh, the patients tend to develop a rather swollen, somewhat tender, upper lip.

The tongue in the *Kali carb.* patient tends to be rather flabby and pale. One associates two types with *Kali carb.* In one there is a thickly coated base, very similar to the *Kali bic.* base. In the other there is a very sensitive, raw tip to the tongue, sometimes with definite blisters on it. These patients often complain of a slimy, flat, bitterish taste in the mouth.

There is some apparent contradiction affecting the appetite. The patients may have complete loss of appetite and an extremely uncomfortable feeling after food; but, if they do not take any food, they develop a very unpleasant, empty, sinking feeling in the abdomen. On the other hand, these patients may have an increased appetite and the only thing that comforts them is a little food taken often; and immediately they become hungry they are uncomfortable again.

As a rule, *Kali carb.* patients have a definite desire for sweet things, actual sugar or sweets, but you will occasionally find—again, an apparent contradiction—a desire for sour things. In most of these cases there is a definite aversion to meat.

In the œsophageal spasm or stricture, the main symptom is a very distressing burning pain behind the middle of the sternum, with a sensation of something hard pressing right through from the front to the back.

When the patients attempt to swallow they have a sensation of the food sticking there, and it may regurgitate into the windpipe, setting up violent spasms of coughing and choking. Associated with the boring pain in the mid-sternum, these patients often complain of a very tender spot in the spine, about the mid-dorsal region between the scapulae.

With reference to their stomach symptoms, one of the most constant *Kali carb.* complaints is a feeling of bloating in the abdomen. This is often accompanied by a sensation of throbbing in the epigastrium, and the whole upper abdomen is exceedingly sensitive to pressure. The sensation of bloating and distension is much worse after any food. With these disturbances, the patients often complain of sharp, stitching pains in the epigastrium, which are very much worse on movement.

Another *Kali carb.* indication is that the patients are liable to have attacks of acute distension during the night, particularly in the early hours of the morning, and their sleep is often seriously disturbed by them.

There is one odd description sometimes given of their abdominal distress. They feel as if the stomach, instead of being distended by wind, were full of water which was sloshing about.

As regards the liver attacks, the usual history given by *Kali carb.* patients is that, after some months of flatulent dyspepsia, they develop recurring slight liver upsets, with sharp stitching pains in the region of the liver, usually extending over to the left side.

Then they begin to have definite rises of temperature—an infective process is taking place. With these temperatures, they are liable to develop a troublesome cough, with acute stitching pains in the right side of the chest and, very often, patches of consolidation in the right lung.

Naturally, they become jaundiced; but, apart from actual acute attacks, you often find *Kali carb.* patients with yellow, scaly patches on the skin, either on the abdomen or on the back. In acute attacks they have a bileless stool; but, quite apart from the acute liver attacks, these patients often complain of a chronic, very light-coloured, painless diarrhœa.

In the majority of cases which I have seen, the *Kali carb.* patients, in spite of chronic indigestion, have been rather overweight than under.

LACHESIS MUTA

THERE are two types of condition that indicate *Lachesis* in abdominal disturbances. The more common is that of the chronic alcoholic; the other is the definitely septic abdomen, and it does not matter whether it is a septic appendix or a septic gall-bladder.

The chronic alcoholic with *Lachesis* indications has certain constant factors. You always get the tremulousness, the congested dusky appearance, the choking sensation round the neck and the desire for air. These chronic alcoholics often complain of exceedingly cold legs and feet—a *Lachesis* indication—and this is often associated with a certain amount of œdema.

As regards the mentality of these alcoholics, in the more acute stage you may find the typical *Lachesis* mentality in which they wander about from one subject to another, and have the difficulty in speech, hurry, impatience and suspicion which you associate with this drug. But much more commonly these patients are in a very phlegmatic, indolent, melancholy state.

Like all chronic alcoholics, they have a typical morning aggravation. They wake with severe nausea, general malaise and weakness, and they steadily improve as the day goes on, often being quite lively in the evenings. When they are feeling horribly heavy and morning-afterish, they are liable to complain of an acute headache on getting up, about the root of the nose, with violent neuralgic pains spreading over the head.

They usually complain of a gnawing sensation in the stomach, which is relieved by food. The way in which the *Lachesis* patient takes his food is sometimes of help—he simply gulps it down. As a rule, after one of these rushed meals, the patient feels horribly bloated and is liable to have violent attacks of belching.

Commonly, the tongue is dry and red, although in the worst cases the tongue develops a brownish streak down the centre. Occasionally I have seen a *Lachesis* alcoholic with a coated tongue and a red streak down the centre, identical with the red streak one associates with *Veratrum viride*.

Lachesis alcoholic gastritis patients have a definite craving for alcohol, and many of them have a craving for oysters—champagne and oysters is the diet of choice. And, of course, any alcohol aggravates their gastric distress.

These patients are liable to have a typical alcoholic liver, with a good deal of general tenderness over the liver and an aggravation from any pressure; they cannot bear any tight clothing. Later, they frequently develop ascites.

In these chronic alcoholics, it is not unlikely that you will find some albuminuria; and a tendency to develop early retinal hæmorrhages, particularly in the left eye, with violent pain and a sensation as if the left eyeball were being squeezed.

Frequently there are recurring attacks of very offensive, putrid smelling diarrhœa.

That is one type of case. The other is the septic abdomen. And here you find the dry, brown tongue more marked than the red. There is likely to be acute thirst; also the thick, difficult speech one tends to associate with *Lachesis*; the difficulty in putting out the tongue, and the marked tremor.

No matter where the sepsis is, whether in the gall-bladder or the appendix, it is always associated with a feeling of intense distension, and it is always accompanied by the most extreme tenderness—these patients can hardly bear to be touched at all, even the least touch on examination being extremely painful.

They complain that they feel as if all the abdominal contents were being twisted up into a tight ball and something would burst.

They tend to have rises of temperature round about 10 o'clock in the evening, and they always feel worse after they have been asleep; they waken feeling poisoned, very often with a violent headache, as if thoroughly drugged from head to foot.

There is one interesting point about their appendix abscesses— or any abscesses down in the right iliac fossa: during the attacks of violent pain, the pain starts in the cæcal region and extends down into the thigh and through into the sacrum on the right side.

In gall-bladder infections, they get exactly the same kind of pain, and it tends to spread across into the stomach, not so much through to the back. In these conditions, they have the same bloated, dusky appearance, the same feeling of general heat, the same desire for air, the feeling that they are being stifled, and very often the same complaint of cold extremities.

If there is any discharge—for instance, in an appendix case after operation—it is always very offensive, the abdominal wound shows no sign of healing at all, and there are dark, unhealthy sloughs, usually associated with a tendency to bleed.

LYCOPODIUM

LYCOPODIUM is one of the common digestive drugs—it is probably more often prescribed for indigestion than any other drug in the materia medica. Almost everyone suffering from flatulence is given *Lycopodium* at some time or other.

Lycopodium patients do suffer from flatulence and you may have indications for it in a simple flatulent dyspepsia, but you will find it frequently indicated in the flatulent dyspepsias associated with some pyloric delay or obstruction, either a simple scarring or a definitely malignant pyloric obstruction.

In most of the cases suffering from flatulent dyspepsia in which *Lycopodium* is well indicated, there is a history of prolonged and intense mental strain for some months preceding the development of the digestive failure. And there are definite *Lycopodium* indications apart from the local conditions.

The *Lycopodium* patient tends to be underweight, many of them are definitely emaciated. They are all tired mentally, finding mental work a great effort; they find themselves making mistakes in routine occupations that they do without thought in the ordinary way; if they go back over their work, they find it is full of mistakes.

Either as a result of this, or independently, they develop a state of timidity, apprehension, general dread and a weak kind of melancholy.

They may show some perverted sensitiveness. They are apt to go to pieces if anyone is kind to them, they break down and may actually weep. But they are equally likely to develop a suspicious, distrustful streak and, if they link this up with their anxiety and general dread, they very often become parsimonious, really from fear rather than from a desire to hoard.

If irritated, *Lycopodium* patients often develop attacks of acute anger, and they always appear to be over-sensitive to pain. Usually they have a sallow complexion, which may be definitely yellowish or yellowish grey; and most typical *Lycopodium* patients I have seen have had a very suggestive yellow discoloration of the teeth.

Frequently their earliest complaints are that they wake up in the morning with a nasty, bitter, dry taste in the mouth, and after meals are liable to have incomplete, unsatisfactory eructations, with a burning sensation in the pharynx and a sour taste in the mouth.

They complain constantly of having a soured stomach and of suffering from attacks of waterbrash, acute acidity, and recurring attacks of hiccough. These attacks of hiccough come on more particularly in the late afternoon or evening, or immediately after a meal.

One constant thing about *Lycopodium* patients is that they are hungry. Even though they are suffering from this feeling of acidity and flatulence, and having constant eructations, they are still hungry and, if they do not have their meals at regular intervals, they are liable to have greater distress.

A meal will often relieve their acidity and, if their meals are delayed, they develop a troublesome, heavy headache. They tell you that frequently they sit down to a meal hungry but feel full up after a few mouthfuls; then the acid eructations start, and they get rid of a quantity of gas and can continue the meal quite comfortably.

They will say that they must eat at regular intervals, otherwise they feel very ill; they have no appetite when they start their delayed meal but, after a few mouthfuls, it returns and they can eat quite a big meal.

All *Lycopodium* patients are aggravated by cold food, and the gastric discomfort is lessened by warm meals. Most of them have a definite desire for sweets which seem to increase the flatulence.

They very often develop an aversion to tobacco, which seems to give them hiccough and increase their acidity; and they often have an aversion to coffee, which also seems to increase their distress.

Quite often they have a liking for starchy foods and an aversion to meat.

With an acute abdominal distension of this type, they are uncomfortable if they have anything tight round their waists, and they dislike all tight clothing.

They complain that they have not only the attacks of acute abdominal distension but also small patches of distension throughout the bowel—localised patches of flatus which are painful for a time, then there is a gurgle and the discomfort disappears. Often they say that by sitting up and rubbing the abdomen, they can shift the flatus on, with almost immediate relief.

The same sort of story is associated with the pyloric obstruction. There is a localised epigastric distension, with definite cramping sensation in the stomach as if it were being squeezed, then there is a gurgle and the whole thing subsides.

With these pyloric obstructions, the patients may feel as if they had a tight cord tied round the upper abdomen and, as the gurgle takes place, the cord seems to slacken off. They also complain of an acute burning pain in the pyloric region.

Most *Lycopodium* patients have a sensation of abdominal weakness: they feel as if the abdominal contents were sagging down, and they want to support the lower abdomen.

Some *Lycopodium* patients suffer from gall-bladder attacks, and may actually develop gallstones. They complain of a constant bruised pain in the hepatic region, and on deep inspiration they get a sharp stitch in the neighbourhood of the gall-bladder.

All *Lycopodium* patients seem to suffer from very obstinate constipation, with which they are liable to develop attacks of acute piles which are extremely painful. But, quite apart from piles, there is often great pain in the anus on attempting to defecate.

Lycopodium cases have a marked aggravation from oysters: you will find it is equally common for *Lycopodium* patients to have a marked desire for oysters, even though they are upset by them.

MAGNESIA CARBONICA

THERE are one or two definite conditions in which there are indications for *Mag. carb.*, the clearest being in cases of acute acid dyspepsia, and like so many patients suffering from this complaint most *Mag. carb.* patients are depressed and very disconsolate. They are aggravated by any mental exertion, particularly by talking.

Frequently they complain that after a good night's sleep, they wake up feeling very weak and worse than before they went to bed. They are always sensitive to noise and to touch. They are also very sensitive to cold, particularly cold draughts, and to any drop in temperature even though it may not become really cold.

Mag. carb. patients are liable to have attacks of acute griping pain associated with violent heartburn, or they may have a feeling of abdominal distension accompanied by acute colic. In these attacks, the abdomen is very sensitive to pressure.

The eructations from which they suffer are either very sour or they are bitter; more commonly, they are sour.

Mag. carb. patients are always aggravated by milk, which seems to sour immediately in their stomachs and increase their distress. They always have a very marked aversion to any green food or green vegetables. Often this is accompanied by a definite liking for meat, which may amount to their taking practically nothing but a meat diet and no vegetables at all, although as a rule they have no aversion to bread and starchy things in general.

The point that makes these patients typically *Mag. carb.* is that, associated with the acid dyspepsia, they are very liable to suffer from either acute facial neuralgia or acute dental neuralgia.

With facial neuralgia, the patient has red-hot shooting pains in the face; which tend to be much worse at night, and the patient finds it impossible to stay in bed and must get up and walk about. They are also very much worse from cold, and from any cold draught.

With dental neuralgia the patient is much worse at night, and very much worse in a warm bed. But, in contrast to the facial ones, these neuralgias are definitely relieved by cold drinks or cold water held in the mouth, whereas the facial ones are very much aggravated by cold in any form.

Mag. carb. patients tend to get their most distressing gastric attacks in the late afternoon, probably between 6 o'clock and 7 o'clock, and they are usually accompanied by nausea. You may confuse this with the *Lycopodium* 4 to 8 aggravation and so miss the *Mag. carb.* indication.

But there are other distinguishing points which help. *Mag. carb.* patients in their attacks of acid dyspepsia, are liable to have colicky pains on the left side of the abdomen or round about the umbilicus:

Lycopodium patients have irregular colicky pains and a sense of general distension.

Following on the attacks of colic, *Mag. carb.* patients have very acute attacks of diarrhœa, usually with green stools which have a very sour smell: practically all *Lycopodium* patients are constipated.

MERCURIUS SOLUBILIS

THERE are two types of condition which indicate *Mercurius*. The first is an acute gastritis; the second is an acute enteritis, either a simple enteritis or one going on to a definite dysentery. In either case there are very definite *Mercurius* indications.

The patients always look ill; they have a very suggestive pale, earthy, puffy appearance, with a moist, sweaty skin. Quite early in the disease, whether it is a gastritis or an enteritis, these *Mercurius* patients become very restless, and very tremulous. Often they have distressing jerking, twitching sensations.

They suffer from troublesome alternations of heat and cold—either becoming intensely hot and unable to bear being covered up, or else pushing off the covers and becoming cold and shivery. But, whether hot or cold, they are sweaty all the time.

With the digestive disturbances, these patients tend to develop troublesome rheumatic pains, which are mostly complained of as bone pains. These become much more troublesome as the patient gets warm, and they are extremely painful as night advances. They are one of the causes of the patient's intense restlessness.

In their attacks of acute gastritis, the patients tend to become definitely apprehensive and worried about themselves. And often rapid in their speech. On the other hand, their mouths become unpleasantly foul, causing difficulty in articulation and they may actually stammer.

In their more serious enteritic conditions, *Mercurius* patients may become very depressed, wretched and miserable. They are rather apt to be distrustful, they feel they are not being properly looked after and are not going to get better. In their wretchedness, when talking about their complaints, they may break down and weep.

The appearance of the *Mercurius* tongue is always very suggestive. The first impression is that it is swollen and toneless, and it has a strange appearance of being somewhat œdematous—it looks watery. With this swollen-looking appearance you may find the imprint of the teeth along the sides.

The tongue is usually palish in colour, but it may have a definite coat, either white or a dirty yellow. A constant characteristic is the peculiar tremulousness of the tongue when it is extruded.

These patients often complain of a very foul or a sweetish taste in the mouth, which is very distressing to them; and always, in all their complaints, they suffer from acute salivation.

In acute gastritis, the patients suffer from extreme burning pain in the pit of the stomach. This is very much aggravated by any food, and is accompanied by extreme heartburn.

Although the pain is aggravated by food, the patients often have a feeling of extreme hunger, frequently accompanied by a craving for stimulants, especially brandy or wine. In these acute gastric upsets, the *Mercurius* patient is always thirsty, and the desire is for cold drinks.

In acute gastritis, *Mercurius* patients may develop acute inflammatory gall-bladder attacks, accompanied by extreme soreness in the region of the liver which is very much aggravated if the patient turns on to the right side. During these attacks, they frequently have a marked nightly aggravation, with rise of temperature, increased discomfort, waves of heat and cold, profuse sweats—a typical septic appearance.

Where there is this type of liver disturbance *Mercurius* patients usually develop an acute aversion to anything fatty or greasy. They also develop an acute aversion to meat of any kind. Associated with the unpleasant sweet taste in the mouth, *Mercurius* patients normally have a marked aversion to sweets.

The enteritis of *Mercurius* is a very violent attack with acute griping pain in the intestine. All the contents of the abdomen feel sore and raw. It is accompanied by a good deal of abdominal distension and very violent tenesmus. The tenesmus is often quite ineffectual and nothing is passed at all. Or there is extremely violent tenesmus and the passage of a very small, bloody mucous stool, accompanied by extreme burning in the rectum.

Not infrequently, with the persistent tenesmus, the patients develop a tendency to very painful rectal prolapse. I recall a number of these acute dysenteries in World War I. It was a bacillary dysentery with severe and almost incessant tenesmus and straining.

As a rule the bowel upset was more marked during the night than during the day. Many of these cases cleared up entirely in a very short time on *Mercurius*.

Depending on the degree of tenesmus and the state of bloodiness of the stools, one prescribed either straight *Mercurius sol.* or else *Mercurius cor.* When the stools contained more blood and less fæcal material, the tenesmus was more violent, and the tendency to prolapse more marked, *Mercurius cor.* gave better results.

MEZEREUM

THERE is a tendency to consider *Mezereum* merely as a skin medicine—for the case with the typical *Mezereum* skin irritation followed by the development of the *Mezereum* rash. But this is one to the very useful medicines for acute gastric ulcer. The ulcer tends to be near the pyloric end of the stomach, but it is definitely a gastric ulcer.

Apart from the pathological condition, there are certain indications which lead one to *Mezereum*. Outstandingly, these gastric patients tend to be hypochondriacal, and their main complaint is that everything feels dead and useless, nothing seems to make a definite, vivid impression. They are depressed and weepy, with a general feeling of dullness, a slight sensation of confusion and a marked forgetful tendency.

As a contrast to their general state, they have spells of irritability and anger, which are characterised by a desire to irritate other people and say something that will vex them.

Their main physical complaint is a general feeling of sickliness, accompanied by a burning sensation in the stomach and a gradually increasing sense of uneasiness. This feeling of discomfort is temporarily relieved by eating. The patients often say that the whole stomach feels raw and that eating makes it more comfortable for the moment.

As a result, *Mezereum* patients often acquire the habit of eating almost continuously, in their desire to relieve their discomfort. Not only is their local condition ameliorated by eating: the patients themselves feel better for it.

There are various contradictions as regards their sensitiveness to heat and cold. The patients as a whole are sensitive to cold air, and yet, when they have the feeling of sickness and nausea, their nausea is aggravated by going into a close room and relieved by going out into the open air. Again, these patients are liable to suffer from acute neuralgic headaches which are definitely aggravated by warmth. It is exactly the same with their eruptions: an irritating eruption is definitely aggravated by warmth and is worse at night, possibly from the warmth of the bed.

The tongue in *Mezereum* tends to be whitely coated, with a sensitive, burning tip. The patients often complain of a peppery taste in the mouth, almost a sensation as if the tongue had been burned, and this burned sensation very often spreads right down the œsophagus into the stomach.

Mezereum patients are very sensitive to any fatty food, which seems to increase their distress. They have a desire for bacon and coffee, and have a definite aversion to meat. As a rule, they are thirsty.

In their gastric upsets, they are very liable to develop attacks of diarrhœa. These attacks are accompanied by rectal tenesmus which, though not severe, is very definite. The stools tend to be sour, watery and undigested. Far more important than the actual appearance of the stool is the sensation of extreme chilliness from which the patient suffers after the bowels have acted.

Mezereum is a very useful drug, and I do not know anything that quite takes its place, and yet it is one that is not very often thought of for this particular condition.

There is one condition, quite apart from its digestive symptoms, in which *Mezereum* is very useful. You will find it extremely helpful for an acute ciliary neuralgia following excision of the eyeball. This is particularly true if the patients get—and many do—a severe sensation of coldness in the eye socket from which the eyeball has been removed. It is quite a common complaint after excision, and is very marked in *Mezereum*, which gives enormous relief in these cases.

NATRUM ARSENICUM

THE majority of instances indicating *Natrum ars.* are cases of definite gastric ulcer, the type of gastric ulcer which is going on to malignancy. As a rule there is a history of the patients being very well nourished, often they have been quite fat; and now they are rapidly losing weight. There is always a feeling on their part that they are seriously ill.

They develop an acute, anxious, nervous kind of restlessness, and very often complain of the feeling that something serious is about to happen to them. With this marked restlessness, they find it quite impossible to settle down to anything, to do any serious work or make any attempt to concentrate.

Natrum ars. patients are always chilly and very sensitive to cold, particularly damp cold. They often get an aggravation from change of weather, particularly a change to wet. In spite of their aggravation from cold, they say that mentally they feel clearer and more alert in the open air; in a stuffy room they become more muddled and find concentration more difficult.

In contrast to their general nervous restlessness, they complain of extreme lassitude, of a sensation of severe weakness, and a very marked aggravation from any exertion—either mental or physical. This sense of tiredness, exaggerated by any exertion, is slightly helped by a meal: food lessens the tired feeling. The appetite may be excessive or there may be a complete aversion to food.

All *Natrum ars.* patients complain of a good deal of flatulence—general abdominal flatulence—and they all suffer from particularly acute gastric pain. The pain may be a general sinking, uncomfortable feeling, a feeling of weight in the epigastrium; or more acute pains, cramping, gnawing, cutting; or just an indefinite feeling of general soreness.

The pain in the stomach usually comes on immediately after food, in spite of the fact that when the condition is not too acute, the patients themselves feel better, less tired and weary, immediately after a meal.

With their digestive upsets, *Natrum ars.* patients develop an acute aggravation from any cold food or drink, either of which increases their discomfort. Any fatty food tends to upset them, and they are particularly aggravated by fruit, milk and pork. Mostly they are aggravated by any alcoholic drink, wine in particular, and especially if it is sour. If they have been in the habit of smoking, they find they develop an acute aversion to their accustomed tobacco, and it seems to increase the gastric discomfort.

They develop a definite desire for sweet things and, occasionally, for bread. They also develop an acute thirst. Very often they have a longing for cold things. But any cold drink or food is apt to produce a sensation of nausea, whereas any hot drink or food tends to increase the stomach pains, particularly the sore, raw feeling.

They have frequent attacks of eructation, with which they bring up a quantity of sourish watery material, and they suffer from almost constant heartburn. As the condition becomes more acute, they get attacks of vomiting; and they may vomit anything—sour mucus, very bitter mucus, bile or blood.

With the tendency to malignancy, there is usually some degree of enlargement of the liver, which is commonly very tender; and the patients are liable to alternating attacks of diarrhœa and constipation.

Natrum ars. patients are more liable to get ulceration on the posterior wall of the stomach; and frequently a severe aching pain going right through to the back, midway between the scapulae. With digestive complaints, they commonly suffer from a degree of urinary frequency, accompanied by difficulty in passing the urine.

These patients often complain bitterly of intensely cold hands and feet. Also of a very troublesome, cold sensation in the back, and they have great difficulty in relieving it. This latter symptom is a useful distinguishing point from *Natrum phos.*, which does not have this sensation of coldness in the back.

Most *Natrum ars.* patients that I have seen have suffered from indefinite rheumatic pains. All have had a degree of skin irritation. In some, the itching has been very troublesome, and in none has it been entirely absent.

Patients requiring one of the sodium salts are liable to suffer from eye strain. The peculiarity of the *Natrum ars.* eye strain is that, where these patients are complaining of pains in or about the eyes, the pains are relieved by warm applications.

I have seen several of these cases where there has been a definite malignant stomach, beyond the operation stage. They have gone downhill quite comfortably on doses of *Natrum ars.* given in low potency. It relieves the greater part of their pain, and I have seen it entirely relieve their vomiting. But they do go downhill in spite of it: it may be that, if one got in earlier, one would be able to cure them, but of that I have no proof.

NATRUM CARBONICUM

THE *Natrum carb.* digestive disturbance is that of a typical flatulent dyspeptic. *Natrum carb.* patients are always complaining of flatulence, heartburn, eructations; and they are acutely conscious of a very spoiled stomach. Usually there is a history of having taken one of the antacid preparations, and of taking it in quite large doses.

It is difficult to place the *Natrum carb.* patient, but I will describe the kind of picture I associate with it.

These patients are usually rather pale, sometimes definitely sallow, with a tendency to yellowish blotches on the skin. They tend to be rather underweight and of poor physique. They very often stand badly with rather stooped shoulders, and give the impression of having a sagging abdomen.

They are always tired-out people; very often with a history of having had a long spell of overwork, and they are exhausted nervously and physically. They complain of inability to work or to concentrate, of a sensation of confusion and a general feeling of brain fag. Most *Natrum carb.* patients are depressed, and occasionally the depression goes on to a definite religious melancholia.

There is always some degree of depression with a dislike of any mental effort. This shows itself in a dislike of meeting strangers or having to talk to people; very often it develops into a dislike of their family, dislike of company in general, and a marked aversion to certain people.

They explain this dislike of certain people in various ways: sometimes they say it is just that they cannot get on with certain people, at other times that certain people exhaust them and leave them dead tired; or simply that they are sensitive to the atmosphere of people.

Natrum carb. people are always nervous, and they have a general trepidation which is very much aggravated by any sudden noise.

If they are startled by a sudden noise they are liable to have definite trembling attacks; they will often get these attacks from excitement of any kind. In addition to being sensitive to noise, most of their senses tend to be over acute; they are over sensitive to light, their sense of taste is over acute. Their sense of smell, too, is always disturbed—sometimes it is over acute but, more commonly, it is entirely absent.

They are always chilly patients, very sensitive to cold, particularly to cold draughts, and yet they are aggravated by extreme heat and are very sensitive to exposure to the sun—they nearly always suffer from sun headaches. They are extremely sensitive to any atmospheric electrical storms.

As regards actual digestive disturbances, they mostly suffer from an acute acid dyspepsia. Their flatulence is greatly aggravated by any starchy food, by vegetables and fatty food. One outstanding point about them is that they have a complete intolerance of milk. It increases the flatulence and is very likely to bring on an attack of diarrhœa.

With the gastric upsets, they always develop an acute thirst, which is liable to be particularly marked after meals.

In spite of the tendency to flatulence after food, they are generally rather more comfortable after eating; but this lasts only for a short time and, a little later, a nasty sinking sensation leads to abdominal pain, general heartburn, flatulence, a feeling of acute distension, probably some colic and later still, a headache may develop.

Natrum carb. patients frequently get a period of extreme hunger late in the evening about 11 p.m., and again in the early morning about 5 a.m. Between 10 a.m. and 11 a.m. they may feel an empty, sinking sensation, but it is not real hunger—the actual hungry periods are more likely to be in the evening, or in the early morning, when the hunger may wake them.

Natrum carb. is very useful in many of the digestive disorders of pregnancy when these are associated with hunger during the night.

Most *Natrum carb.* patients are constipated but in acute digestive upsets they occasionally get an attack of violent diarrhœa, which is usually greyish and watery, very sudden in its onset and difficult to control. The *Natrum carb.* patients who tend to have these recurring attacks of diarrhœa may also have a certain amount of enlargement of the liver, and be slightly jaundiced.

All *Natrum carb.* patients tend to suffer from recurring attacks of catarrh in various situations: it may be a recurring leucorrhœa, a recurring nasal discharge, or an old otitis. The constant characteristic about these catarrhs is that, no matter where they are situated, they are always accompanied by very thick yellow discharges.

All the *Natrum carb.* patients I have seen have had diffuse rheumatic pains; complaining of creaking sensations in the cervical region, pains in their backs, weakness of the ankles and sensitiveness of the soles of the feet.

They all tend to have very dry skins, and they frequently complain of painful, dry cracks on the fingers, particularly the finger-tips, and of the same sort of thing on the toes.

Many of these patients, in spite of their general emaciation or loss of weight, get œdema about the ankles in the evenings, when they are tired.

They are all susceptible to herpetic attacks. They get eruptions round about the hair, they may get herpetic patches on the lips, and are liable—particularly the older patients—to suffer from attacks of thrush. Thrush in old women not infrequently requires *Natrum carb.* For children with milk upsets and milk diarrhœa accompanied by thrush, *Natrum carb.* is one of the biggest standbys.

The drug that is most commonly confused with *Natrum carb.* is *Sepia*, and many of the patients who appear to need *Sepia* really require *Natrum carb.*

NATRUM MURIATICUM

IT is not easy to ascertain from the textbooks the *Natrum mur.* type of digestive upset. In acute cases most of them have either an acute gastritis or a gastric ulcer. Some *Natrum mur.* patients have a chronic colitis, with a somewhat enlarged liver and general abdominal discomfort and diarrhœa; but that is a much more chronic condition.

I have not found any record in textbooks that *Natrum mur.* subjects had anything suggestive of a gastric ulcer, and yet in practice I have met it quite frequently, with definite ulceration shown by X-ray, and vomiting of blood, either bright red or coffee-ground vomit; but there is no record of this in the materia medica. In these cases, one prescribes neither on the local condition, nor on the digestive symptoms, but on the fact that the patient is a *Natrum mur.* subject.

The only way to tackle the problem is to consider the characteristics of the *Natrum mur.* patient and the pathological conditions which have responded to it.

It is easy to be misled by the textbook statement that *Natrum mur.* patients tend to be emaciated. Experience shows that they may be rather thin about the face and neck, but are surprisingly well nourished from the waist downwards: they very often have quite fat thighs and hips, and quite solid legs and feet. They tend to have a rather greasy skin and this is much aggravated during meal times; they break out in a greasy sweat when eating.

Most of them have a relative anæmia. It may not be very obvious because they tend to flush easily, but when the flush settles you find there is a definite pallor; they usually have a lowish red cell count. Most of them have rather pale mucous membranes.

The most important thing about the typical *Natrum mur.* mentality is its instability. The patients are either very depressed, terrified and miserable, or else they are over-excited, very bright, very often laughing; and they tend to swing from one mood to the other. They are always rather emotional, intense types, and are aggravated by any excitement.

All their senses tend to be over acute. They are oversensitive to noise. Though they are not quite so sensitive to thunder as the

Natrum carb. patients, they are very definitely sensitive to it, and liable to get thunder headaches. They are emotionally acutely sensitive to music. They cannot stand being ignored. They very definitely like attention, and yet dislike expressed sympathy; it annoys them and may make them cry.

Mentally, they are somewhat tired; rather absent-minded; tend to be forgetful and any extreme mental effort is liable to produce a headache.

When a *Natrum mur.* patient complains of headaches from mental effort, it is always worthwhile having his eyes tested, because many *Natrum mur.* patients suffer from eye strain. Morning headaches in *Natrum mur.* are much more likely to be due to an ocular defect than anything else, and very often clear up with the aid of a pair of glasses even without the administration of *Natrum mur.*

Occasionally after a dose of *Natrum mur.* there is a definite improvement in vision without glasses—the headaches disappear, also the sensation of eye strain, but the majority will require glasses before their headaches can be cured.

It is not usual to find a real *Natrum mur.* patient who has not been subject to headaches; and their headaches are particularly bad, and extremely severe in character. It is usually a throbbing headache, and the patient wakes up with it in the morning; it tends to get worse all day, and does not disappear until after a night's sleep.

There is another type of *Natrum mur.* headache which develops a little after getting up, or during the earlier part of the forenoon, and tends to clear again about sunset. These headaches are brought on by any excitement or over-work, and occur very often about the menstrual period. They are, in fact, often periodic in nature quite apart from menstruation.

They are often brought on by railway journeys. They may go on to definite attacks of sickness and vomiting. Another thing that will always produce the *Natrum mur.* headache is irregularity in meals. If the *Natrum mur.* patient is accustomed to lunch at 1 o'clock and has to go on to 2 o'clock or half-past, he is very apt to develop a headache, which will then not subside until he has had a night's rest. This is a question of tiredness more than anything else.

All these patients are sensitive to heat, particularly to hot, stuffy atmospheres. They are worse in a warm room and better in the open air. They are very uncomfortable if they get overheated in any way—from over-exertion, stuffy atmosphere, too much excitement; and yet, many of their complaints are better for gentle, reasonable exercise which does not make them hot.

Practically all *Natrum mur.* patients suffer from headache, constipation, or both, on going to the seaside. Very often this corrects itself in a week or so. Although the headaches may correct themselves, you will find quite a number of these patients who say that, while they enjoy the seaside, they have a headache all the time they are there: it is never severe, but it is constant, and you will find that all these cases suffer from either acute or relative constipation throughout their stay.

As far as the actual digestive symptoms are concerned, there are one or two suggestive points. First of all, the *Natrum mur.* patients suffer from two types of tongue. They all tend to get herpetic eruptions about the mouth, particularly if they catch a cold, and they may get small ulcers on the lips and tongue. But the typical *Natrum mur.* tongue is rather coated, with clear areas as if the coating had been stripped off in patches producing a mapped appearance. This is the most typical *Natrum mur.* tongue. The other is a very shiny, red tongue which tends to have small frothy patches of saliva down the sides.

As regards the appetite, *Natrum mur.* patients tend to get very hungry in the middle of the morning—there is a typically *Natrum mur.* empty, sinking sensation between 10 and 11 a.m. Quite distinct from this, they very often have an exceedingly good appetite. They usually have a liking for definitely bitter food, sour things and salt food. Often they have a definite craving for starchy food, and a strong liking for milk and fish. Occasionally, you come across a *Natrum mur.* patient who has a passion for oysters.

In their gastric upsets, they develop an acute aversion to bread, to fat of any kind, rich foods in general and to meat. They sometimes have an aversion to coffee, and there is the statement that the *Natrum mur.* patient has an aversion to tobacco. I am not convinced of this since you find the *Natrum mur.* patient who has an acute aversion to tobacco when it is smoked by one person and no aversion at all when it is smoked by another. But, it is laid down in the textbooks that *Natrum mur.* patients have an aversion to tobacco.

One of the common complaints made in connection with their digestion is a feeling of a lump in the throat. It may be just a feeling of discomfort, in which case, after a little eructation, the whole thing disappears. There may, however, be actual difficulty in swallowing, and you will sometimes meet a *Natrum mur.* patient who, on swallowing, has definite pain at the cardiac entrance of the stomach.

They make the complaint that they have a feeling of a lump in the stomach after food, a feeling of general fullness and discomfort.

Quite frequently they complain of what they describe as acute "ulcerative pain"—it is an acute burning pain really, but one quite frequently gets the description that they have the feeling that they have an ulcer in the stomach.

With their more acute gastric upsets, they are liable to get attacks of vomiting, the vomiting usually being rather difficult; and the vomit itself consisting of white, slimy mucus which may be bloodstained. The vomiting always gives a marked sensation of relief. In acute gastric upsets, these patients always tend to be thirsty.

X-ray frequently shows these patients suffering from definite gastric ulcer at the cardiac end or on the lesser curvature, and I do not remember a *Natrum mur.* patient with a duodenal or pyloric ulcer.

Most *Natrum mur.* patients suffer from constipation, but you sometimes get patients with a chronic diarrhœa. In these, there is a constant complaint of a horrid, dragging sensation in the abdomen; it feels as if everything was sagging down, and they do get a certain amount of comfort from external abdominal support. With these chronic diarrhœas, there is usually some degree of hepatic enlargement: in dealing with an old malarial patient, there may be some degree of splenic enlargement, too.

After the 1914-18 War, I saw quite a number of men who had been out East and had chronic malaria. They came back suffering from what was really a malarial diarrhœa—at least, a chronic diarrhœa dating from recurring attacks of malaria. The diarrhœa was very nondescript in character. It cleared up very well on *Natrum mur.* All of them had a degree of enlargement of the liver, and some splenic enlargement too: the spleens subsided materially after *Natrum mur.*

All *Natrum mur.* patients suffer from very irritating skin eruptions. It may be nothing more than an urticaria, or it may go on to a definite vesicular eruption. The eruption may occur on any part of the body. There is no doubt that the urticarial ones are associated with digestive upsets while the more herpetic ones are not.

Also a constant factor in *Natrum mur.* patients is their invariable complaint of a sensation of dryness in all their mucous membranes. Their lips feel dry, their mouths feel dry, very often they complain of a hot dry throat; and it is quite common for these patients to suffer from a chronic atrophic pharyngitis.

They are mostly susceptible to acute colds, acute coryzas, and they may have a susceptibility to acute attacks of hay fever. The discharge of all the mucous membranes of *Natrum mur.* is white—a white, stringy discharge just like white of egg. This is a distinguishing point from *Natrum carb.*, in which the discharges are yellow.

NATRUM PHOSPHORICUM

FROM the materia medica descriptions of *Natrum phosphoricum* and *Natrum arsenicum* it is practically impossible to distinguish one from the other. If one notes the symptoms of the two drugs as recorded in the materia medica, one finds they are practically identical.

Natrum phos. does not usually have the history of extremely rapid loss of weight which is associated with *Natrum ars.*, nor have the patients been very much overweight to begin with. On the whole, there is rather more mental prostration in *Natrum phos.* than in *Natrum ars.*, and there is not the same degree of nervous, restless anxiety.

Natrum phos. patients are very tired, and they feel that talking is a dreadful effort. There may be a certain amount of bashfulness in *Natrum phos.* which is not commonly met with in *Natrum ars.* Rather than the inability to concentrate of *Natrum ars.*, there is liable to be extreme forgetfulness in *Natrum phos.* Rather than the typical *Natrum ars.* fear of something going wrong with them physically, the *Natrum phos.* patient tends to get a sensation of something unpleasant going to happen, particularly during the night.

Another pointer to the selection of *Natrum phos.* is that the patient is very likely to suffer from headaches after any mental effort—a symptom which is not so noticeable in *Natrum ars.*

In both drug pictures there is a great sensitivity to cold, but there is none of the mental relief in the open air in *Natrum phos.* that you find in *Natrum ars.*: in fact, *Natrum phos.* is very sensitive to the open air or to draughts, and very liable to take cold from any draught of air or change of temperature.

Both have very much the same feeling of general weakness and an aggravation from exertion. Both are more tired and exhausted when they are hungry, and rather better after a meal.

In *Natrum phos.* there is rather more general sensitiveness. They are more sensitive to noise and to music; more sensitive to their surroundings, and more aggravated by electrical storms than the *Natrum ars.* patients.

So far as the foods which upset them are concerned, the two drugs are identical. They are both upset by fats, cold food or drink, milk, fruit, sour things of any kind—sour wine, fruit, drinks.

Their desires have some distinguishing points. *Natrum phos.* patients often develop a definite desire for alcohol and for highly tasting food. Sometimes there is a desire for eggs and for fried fish. Both of them have a desire for cold drinks, but the aggravation from cold foods—the nausea following them—seems more marked in *Natrum ars.* than in *Natrum phos.*

Another helpful point: most *Natrum phos.* patients have a very thick, yellow coating to the base of the tongue. At times they complain of a horrible sensation as if they had a hair on the soft palate or on the tongue, which causes acute irritation.

A complaint from which *Natrum phos.* patients are likely to suffer is a definite ulceration in the stomach, associated with a good deal of acid dyspepsia and flatulence. And, as in *Natrum ars.*, they are liable to suffer from alternating attacks of diarrhœa and constipation. There is less likely to be an actual hæmatemesis in *Natrum phos.*: but more likely a sour mucous vomit.

In many of these cases, when the patient is hungry, there is a very empty sensation which is not relieved by eating. Not infrequently you hear the report that they develop a gnawing epigastric pain which comes on about two hours after a meal.

In contrast with the generalised irritation of the skin found in *Natrum ars.*, in *Natrum phos.* there is liable to be a very irritating, localised eruption round about the ankles. Both complain bitterly of intense coldness of hands and feet but *Natrum phos.* cases do not complain of the coldness of the back of the *Natrum ars.* patient and there is not the pain between the scapulae.

Male *Natrum phos.* patients are very liable to suffer from extremely exhausting, recurring emissions.

NATRUM SULPHURICUM

THE most common condition requiring *Natrum sulph.* is that which used to be called a sluggish liver. The patients have a very slow digestion, and can digest only the simplest types of food. They suffer a lot from nausea, particularly after any farinaceous food, and are liable to attacks of bilious vomiting, usually associated with a good deal of abdominal colic.

The mouth feels horribly slimy, and there is always a dirty tongue —a dirty, greyish, greenish, slimy tongue—and a very bitter taste in the mouth. There is a very definite aversion to bread and meat, and usually a marked thirst for cold drinks.

This typical condition, occurring in a patient who is very sensitive to heat, very much worse in warm weather, liable to attacks of this type coming on in the spring, aggravated by damp, and who is definitely better in the open air, better when moving about, worse when at rest, and who has the peculiar mentality of *Natrum sulph.* will respond to this drug every time.

The characteristic state of these patients is one of depression. They feel heavy, they do not want to be disturbed, they do not want to be spoken to, and they cannot be bothered to speak. There is a general feeling of dislike of everything, and this may go on to an acute loathing of life, almost a melancholic state. But in spite of the tendency to turn their faces to the wall and give up the struggle, there is a streak of anxiety about themselves running through their outlook.

Their depression is very marked, and it is aggravated by music. It is usually very marked in the morning on waking, and tends to improve after breakfast, i.e. after some food; and it is definitely relieved after stool.

In spite of their general sluggishness, *Natrum sulph.* patients are always over-sensitive to pain. And they have a peculiarly extreme sensitiveness to light. In acute conditions, they want their room darkened and to be left in peace; it is astonishing how often you find a *Natrum sulph.* patient lying with his back to the room.

With liver upsets, they very quickly acquire a slightly jaundiced tinge. It may be an extreme jaundice, and, in acute attacks, they are prone to develop vesicles, particularly on the lower lip.

The attack may be a simple catarrhal jaundice, with enlarged, tender liver—very sensitive to pressure; or it may be a definitely enlarged gall-bladder with gall-stones and gall-stone colic. But, no matter which it is, there is the same description of the discomfort they feel below the right costal margin—that is to say, they get pain and tenderness on lying on the right side, owing to the pressure on the liver. They also get a dragging sensation if they lie on the left side, due to the drag of the congested liver.

Such is the most likely type of attack which the *Natrum sulph.* patients are liable to suffer. Usually with these bilious attacks, they suffer from very severe occipital headache, often with the sensation that the head is being dragged back on to the pillow.

Another condition to which *Natrum sulph.* patients are prone is a fairly acute attack of appendicitis, with extreme pains in the cecal region. Apparently, it is a retro-cecal appendix, because they always complain of extreme pain going right round to the back, rather than of pain over McBurney's Point. It is the type of appendix which is associated with a degree of jaundice.

Some of the most striking results from *Natrum sulph.* have been in cases of appendix abscesses, where there has been a retro-cecal appendix and a tendency for the inflammation to track up and conditions suggesting a sub-phrenic.

I have never seen a definite sub-phrenic abscess cleared up with *Natrum sulph.*, but I have seen several cases in which there was a definite tracking inflammation going up under the liver, with a nasty swinging temperature. Cases which had been operated on and were obviously going downhill, and in which there was a tendency to involvement of the chest, particularly the left lower lobe; and they have cleared up in the most astonishing way on *Natrum sulph.*

In the ordinary acute appendix, in addition to the locality of the pain and the general make-up of the patient, one constant is a very troublesome urging to stool, which merely results in the passage of a quantity of flatus. The other characteristic with these appendix cases is a very troublesome, gushing diarrhœa, accompanied by acute cramping pain in the abdomen. This is liable to be very marked first thing in the morning, immediately the patient gets out of bed.

Concurrently with the attack—be it liver, gall-bladder or appendix—the patients are very liable to get a suppurative condition about the root of the nails. I have verified this several times. A patient with a chronic liver who, with a slight increase of digestive disturbance always develops suppurating places round his nails, will very often need *Natrum sulph.*

There is one other rather interesting point about this remedy, and it has no connection with the digestive system. *Natrum sulph.* is sometimes very well indicated in acute hip joints, particularly when it is the right hip which is affected. The pain is very similar in character to that experienced in cases of appendicitis, and if there are any *Natrum sulph.* indications, it is worthwhile to consider its use. Two cases in hospital cleared up remarkably well on *Natrum sulph.*, and it is apt to be forgotten for this condition.

NITRICUM ACIDUM

THERE are one or two conditions in which *Nitricum acidum* is particularly useful from the digestive point of view, far and away the commonest of which is ulceration of the lower bowel.

You seldom get indications for this remedy in an ordinary acute gastritis, except in a typical *Nitricum acidum* patient. But the kind of case in which you get indications for it is the very old, broken-down, chronic ill-health patient, very often with an old digestive history dating back over years, with indefinite bouts of diarrhœa.

Often there is a history of an old dysentery or something similar; and the patient complains of indefinite abdominal discomfort, very often with pains centred round the right iliac fossa. It is not clear whether the patient has a chronic appendix or whether it is a legacy from an old dysentery with a chronically inflamed cæcum and a history of recurring diarrhœa which is always very painful.

The other type is the patient with a history of tuberculosis. He is liable to get feverish attacks with an irregular, swinging temperature, and sweating; associated with that, he has digestive disturbances, again with recurring attacks of diarrhœa.

In addition to this pathological background the *Nitricum acidum* picture is important. As a rule, the patient is somewhat emaciated, easily tired, and always in a very nervy, excitable, irritable, peevish condition. The irritability may be very acute and go on to violent attacks of rage, or it may be a general peevishness tending towards despondency and hopelessness, with some degree of anxiety.

Nitricum acidum patients are usually dark-complexioned and rather swarthy; usually they have brown hair and brown eyes. They are very easily startled; they jump at noises or at any sudden approach, and they are particularly liable to be scared if anyone suddenly touches them. Another common feature in the *Nitricum acidum* patient is a red nose.

The *Nitricum acidum* picture is of someone looking rather thin, dark and sallow, with a very red nose. Most of these patients complain that their noses often get blocked, and they commonly suffer from a persistent post-nasal discharge.

These patients usually suffer from severe headaches, whose type is most suggestive. There is always a sensation of increased tension in the head: the patients describe it either as feeling like something clamping down on the head, or else as a constricting, tight band round the head.

They are always very sensitive to cold; they are chilly patients, and cold aggravates all their complaints.

They commonly have an unhealthy mouth. There are small exceedingly sensitive blisters on the tongue and on the inside of the cheeks; and the gums become inflamed with a good deal of bleeding and a very offensive smell. There is always considerable salivation and, nearly always, a tendency to develop cracks at the angles of the lips.

As regards the actual digestive condition, the *Nitricum acidum* patient is very much upset by milk, which produces a sour eructation and a feeling of intense bitterness. The patient very often gets this bitter taste after any food, and quite often he gets eructations tasting of what he has eaten many hours before.

In spite of these digestive upsets, *Nitricum acidum* patients often have a ravenous hunger, but are particularly uncomfortable after a meal. They develop an acute craving for highly-tasting food—salt, pickled herring, etc. Often they have a strange desire for fat; and yet any fatty food is very liable to produce a sensation of nausea.

In all their conditions, these patients have a definite aversion to meat and to bread. They say the bread turns sour and is liable to produce sickness and vomiting.

These patients very often feel more comfortable while they are actually eating; afterwards, they get the burning sensation in the stomach which goes on to definite abdominal colic. During the period of discomfort, the *Nitricum acidum* patients feel very hot and sweaty.

There are two characteristic conditions in connection with the stomach. One is on swallowing when there is a feeling of obstruction at the cardiac end of the stomach. There may actually be acute stitching pain in that region on swallowing, and occasionally X-ray reveals a definite lesion. More commonly it is merely a spasm, but there may be actual ulceration.

The other condition is a similar spasm in the pyloric region; on palpation in the epigastrium there is very often a tender spot over the pylorus. Where this is present in addition to sour eructations after food, the patients are liable to develop nausea and vomiting; they frequently vomit a quanity of tenacious, bloody mucus, which is very offensive.

In the abdomen, there are attacks of colic with severe pinching, stitching pains, and a complaint of constant abdominal disturbances, a feeling of rumbling in the abdomen which the patients very often describe as if their inside were boiling. These attacks of abdominal pain may come on some little time after a meal, or they may be induced by the patient's being exposed to cold.

With the more chronic abdominal disturbance, *Nitricum acidum* patients get a certain amount of enlargement—congestion—of the liver, and there may be a degree of jaundice.

The most common characteristic is the liability to attacks of diarrhœa. The actual character of the stool varies very much with the pathological condition, but it is always very offensive. It may contain mucus or blood. On examination, there is very likely to be a definite—possibly very extensive—ulceration in the rectum.

From experience, I have not found *Nitricum acidum* helpful in carcinoma of the rectum. One would think it should help because it has the symptoms—the pain, the urging, the offensive stools and the blood and mucus, but I have never seen it do much good. It seems to have more affinity for an ulcerative colitis.

The constant characteristic of *Nitricum acidum* diarrhœa is its extreme painfulness. The patients get colicky attacks before stool, and they get an extremely severe tenesmus during stool and after: in fact, it is even worse after the passage of the motion than during it. They describe it as if the rectum were being torn, or as if knives were sticking into it. You will see them simply writhing in agony.

In addition to the offensiveness, the *Nitricum acidum* stool is very excoriating. I have seen cases with extensive excoriation spreading right back between the buttocks, the whole area being extremely painful.

There is a tendency, as would be expected with this enlarged liver and the bowel irritation, for *Nitricum acidum* patients to suffer from piles. These indications for *Nitricum acidum* appear mostly in a patient who for some time, has had piles which have had a tendency to bleed but have never been very troublesome; then, for some reason, the bleeding has suddenly stopped and the piles have become inflamed and intensely painful, especially after the bowels have acted.

This, in the typical, broken-down kind of patient in which *Nitricum acidum* is indicated, is the case that responds very well.

In addition to piles, with the chronic diarrhœa these patients are very liable to develop fissures about the anus. These are extremely tender, very sensitive to touch and often burn like fire. Patients say when the bowels act, it feels as if the fissure were being split open, or as if it were being cut by a knife.

There is one other point about *Nitricum acidum* patients which is almost constant: they tend to have a very strong-smelling urine. It is almost as penetrating as the BENZOICUM ACIDUM urine, and has very much the same character, often described as "horse's urine"

There is one weird thing about *Nitricum acidum* patients. Certain of their symptoms are produced, or aggravated, by railway travel. They are liable to get a headache from it, and to get sick; and yet, certain of their other disturbances are definitely helped by travelling—even their headache is sometimes relieved by it.

Occasionally you find a patient who says that the only time he is comfortable is when travelling. You may get it either way: travelling may relieve them or it may aggravate them. So, if you get a patient who says travelling always does him good, do not rule out *Nitricum acidum*. The common thing is for the *Nitricum acidum* patient to be aggravated by travelling of any kind, but you will occasionally come across patients on whom it has the opposite effect.

NUX MOSCHATA

INDICATIONS for this drug will be found in three different conditions. First, in old people in whom there is very obstinate constipation; the bowels do not seem to act on any provocation at all. Second, in the somewhat hysterical woman who has been having rather profuse periods which have been suddenly checked. Third, in certain emotional disturbances in pregnancy. The constant feature in all three states is that the patients all feel as if the abdomen were blown out almost to bursting point.

Where these conditions appear together with the indications for *Nux moschata*, there is a very definite, clear-cut picture.

Associated with the local condition, is the strange mental picture of *Nux moschata*. It is a strange state of almost bewilderment. The patients complain of all sorts of strange sensations all over. They cannot remember things properly, have a horrible feeling of weakness, feel as if any effort was an enormous labour, and they are liable to complain of general aching all over as if they had over-exerted themselves.

They also complain of a constant faint, sickly sort of feeling, and an overpowering sense of sleepiness. That is the constant state of all three types of patient. But the rather hysterical, suppressed menstrual patient and the pregnancy patient with the mild mental disturbance are liable to get periods in which suddenly everything strikes them as perfectly ludicrous; they burst out laughing in hysterical attacks of laughter which are quite likely to go on to attacks of weeping.

All these patients complain that their memory has gone to pieces and they cannot remember anything.

They complain of their mouths being incredibly dry, which is very distressing to them. Their tongue sticks to the roof of their mouth. It is not a feeling of thirst—they are not at all thirsty—but they will hold anything juicy in their mouths in order to relieve this horrible feeling of dryness. The condition is liable to be most troublesome in the morning on waking.

Practically all *Nux moschata* patients have a very large appetite, and usually they are very fast eaters. They complain that after a meal it feels as if the food remained in hard lumps in the stomach, producing a sensation of extreme soreness.

With the attacks of abdominal distension, there is a certain amount of nausea which may be quite acute; and pregnancy patients are liable to suffer from very severe morning sickness—intense nausea in the morning whenever they raise their heads off the pillow. With the general abdominal disturbance, they get a sensation as if diarrhœa were just about to start. They do have attacks of diarrhœa—a very sudden, profuse diarrhœa, followed by the sensation of abdominal distension which still persists.

The older people, after an attack of diarrhœa, are liable to develop very obstinate constipation. With this they feel so distended that they feel they will actually burst something if it is not relieved.

In addition to the local disturbances, there are one or two other pointers to *Nux moschata*. For instance, these patients, who are very chilly, very often complain of a sensation of extreme coldness of the skin and extreme dryness. They practically never perspire, and the sensation of dryness applies not only to the skin but to all the mucous membranes. They are always very sensitive to exposure to cold air, particularly to cold wind and if they come into a warmish room after being out in the cold air, they will sit down and go to sleep at once. This tendency is extreme in *Nux moschata* patients.

If they are walking against a wind, particularly a cold one, they are very liable to become breathless, and are quite liable to suffer from loss of voice after exposure to cold air. Quite apart from this loss of voice due to exposure to cold, they also have a tendency to get hysterical aphonia which usually comes on after any emotional disturbance.

There is one other peculiar disturbance to which they tend. With their mental bewilderment, they complain that everything seems far too big. It is a visual disturbance, it is the things they look at that seem too big. Even their own hands, when they look at them, appear to be double the size they ought to be. It is not everyone who sees things bigger than they ought to be who needs *Platinum*; occasionally, they need a dose of *Nux moschata*.

NUX VOMICA

FOR the ordinary acute attack of indigestion due to an indiscretion in diet, *Nux* is almost a specific, especially if the indiscretion has been particularly marked. Time and again, when a patient who has had a large and too rich dinner with alcoholic liquor to wash it down, takes a dose of *Nux*—quite low potency—before going to bed, he will get up next morning feeling perfectly well instead of liverish, headachy and bad-tempered.

Similarly on the day after the indiscretion, when they are feeling absolutely rotten. There is the common *Nux* story of sleeplessness during the greater part of the night, particularly round about 3 a.m. (the usual *Nux* sleepless period), and then falling asleep about 7 a.m. when they should be getting up. It was extremely difficult to wake when it was time to get up, and they have a beastly head, a foul taste in the mouth, feel sickish and are generally off colour. That is the common *Nux* story, and a dose of *Nux* will wipe out the whole thing in twenty minutes or half an hour.

When this acute picture is firmly understood, it gives also the key to the chronic *Nux* case. The patient who has been persistently overdoing it—and the overdoing need not necessarily be a dietetic error, it may be overwork, too much anxiety, too much stress—can get into very much the same state. He has disturbed nights, does not sleep well, and then, falling into a heavy sleep in the latter part of the night, awakes feeling perfectly awful when it is time to get up.

One of the outstanding *Nux* characteristics is that the patients say they have the feeling that if only they could vomit they would be better. It does not matter whether that feeling arises in the course of an acute digestive attack or in a chronic condition, the statement is always the same: the patients say they feel as if their stomachs were loaded up. In actual fact, they are better immediately after they have vomited.

Another constant factor is that the process of vomiting is very difficult. They retch and strain, and then bring up a quantity of material which is very bitter, sour and scalding. Added to this mighty effort of vomiting is the *Nux* characteristic disturbance of peristaltic movement. It occurs throughout the whole of the hollow viscera.

The patients are liable to be very constipated and any effort seems to increase their constipation. They have intense straining to get their bowels to act. When they do act, there is the feeling that the action is incomplete—it feels as if there were some stool left behind—and the patients go on straining to try to expel this; and the more straining they do, the greater the spasm of the sphincter.

There is exactly the same kind of disturbance in connection with the bladder. There is extreme difficulty in passing urine, and the more effort made the more difficulty there is; if the patients just wait quietly, the urine flows away but if they make an effort, the sphincter seems to close down and they cannot pass urine at all.

This is the general description of the kind of digestive upsets the *Nux* patients get. The condition may go further. With the history of overdoing things in a dietetic way, they are apt to get a good deal of congestion of the liver. There may even be definite enlargement of the liver with a constant feeling of distension in the upper abdomen; and actual attacks of jaundice and even the development of gall-stones, with acute hepatic colic.

The *Nux* make-up is typical and these patients either are, or tend to be, rather underweight. They are a highly nervous type, and are very much strung up. They are very irritable, and liable to fly into a rage; they are hard to please, touchy and extremely difficult to satisfy either in business or at home—conditions are never quite right for them. Occasionally, in extreme states, you get a patient who is definitely malicious and spiteful. No *Nux* patient can stand contradiction.

That is the typical case, but occasionally you come across a *Nux* patient who does not appear to be so much on wires, who is much more quiet and sullen, and very definitely dislikes being spoken to; he is rather surly and has an aversion to doing anything or talking at all. It is not the type associated with *Nux*, but I have seen such cases. In dealing with this type of patient, *Nux* helps them up to a point but you have to follow up with *Sepia*.

Typical *Nux* patients are exceedingly sensitive to any external impressions. They are very sensitive to noise, smell, light, music and, especially, to pain.

As regards particular foods, *Nux* patients are liable to be upset by any very rich food. They are upset by coffee, tea, stimulants and tobacco; and very much upset by over-eating. You will find that, if the typical *Nux* patient is worried or chivvied about, his digestion is at once affected and he cannot digest his food.

So far as desires for food are concerned, *Nux* patients always have a craving for something with a marked taste—some definitely stimulating type of food—although it makes their digestion worse. They do not really mind what the food is, so long as it has a bite about it.

As a rule, these patients complain of a nasty feeling of distension which sometimes comes on immediately after a meal but more usually two or three hours after food. The distension is so extreme that they have to loosen their clothes, and it is very often accompanied by acute colicky abdominal pains. With these colicky pains coming on as digestion proceeds, there is often a typical *Nux* sudden urging to stool.

Another common *Nux* characteristic: while having a good meal—particularly one of their favourite stimulating meals—the ordinarily pale *Nux* patients are liable to flush up, become hot and sweaty. Often after a meal, they are very sleepy and heavy.

Nux patients need a sound night's sleep. The *Nux* condition may develop due to the fact that the patient has not been having good nights, either from stress or worry; and you will find that any persistent loss of sleep is liable to produce the definite *Nux* condition. One of the difficulties of these patients is that under conditions of stress they become sleepless. When they are sleepless, any noise in the neighbourhood is enough to keep them awake; or they just lie awake and worry about their daily business.

All *Nux* patients are intensely chilly and very sensitive to cold—cold draughts, cold air. They feel miserable in cold weather, and are apt to become much more irritable if chilled. Yet, in spite of their acute chilliness, many become faint in a hot, stuffy atmosphere.

There is one strange *Nux* condition which does not appear to indicate *Nux* at all: during a very good meal, particularly if accompanied by a good deal of alcohol and eaten in a very hot room, *Nux* patients sometimes develop acute gastric distension. They get a feeling of severe gastric oppression, as if their clothes were too tight, accompanied by acute abdominal colic; a feeling as if they were going to have violent diarrhœa, and followed by a sensation of extreme faintness.

Remember, therefore, that a diner who becomes rather dusky, has obvious abdominal flatulence, is growing faint and wants to loosen his clothes, does not necessarily need *Carbo veg*. Many need *Nux* which acts much more quickly, is almost instantaneous, and in a moment or two the patient becomes perfectly comfortable.

Sometimes there are indications for *Nux* in ordinary pregnancy morning sickness, particularly if it is associated with the typical *Nux* sleeplessness. It is a very nondescript morning nausea with headache. When this is associated with the typical *Nux* constipation—the feeling that the bowels are never completely emptied—it will very often control the morning sickness, even in patients who are not typically *Nux*.

The *Nux* type of constipation is often stressed, but the cases do suffer from very troublesome diarrhœa as well. It is a very painful, colicky diarrhœa, and the characteristic thing is the actual stool. There is great urging to stool, the passage of the stool is very difficult, and the stool consists of a quantity of water in which there are a number of hard lumps usually covered with mucus and it appears to be a case of acute irritation superimposed on a chronic constipation.

OPIUM

THERE are various points in *Opium* which are very interesting and which make a striking contrast with *Nux vomica*. It has very many of the symptoms which one associates with *Nux*—for instance, the severe morning headache, the nausea, the loss of appetite and the dislike of getting up. Occasionally these are indications for *Opium* in people who have had a really bad debauch and have been completely "blotted out" the night before. It is a more extreme stage than the ordinary gastric upset from an indiscretion which one associates with *Nux*.

These, however, are not the conditions for which one ordinarily thinks of *Opium* in digestive disturbances. The outstanding feature is complete, or almost complete, obstruction somewhere in the digestive canal, usually in the bowel. There are very clear indications in different pathological conditions associated with obstruction and obstructive vomiting.

The condition which most commonly calls for *Opium* is paralytic ileus after an abdominal section. There is a loop of bowel which is completely paralysed, accompanied by reversed peristalsis and the pumping of bile back into the stomach. The patient vomits violently, bringing up masses of bile-stained, rather foul-smelling vomit, and has an extreme sensation of abdominal distension. This is the commonest condition in which *Opium* is most useful.

It is very interesting to note that in the majority of cases of a paralytic ileus, there is a history that opium, or one of its derivatives, has been given before or after the operation.

Another condition frequently indicating *Opium* is intussusception in children. Again, there is intestinal obstruction with spasmodic intestinal contractions, colicky attacks, extreme urging, and the passage of nothing but a little blood-stained mucus. Later, there is vomiting, first of bile and then of fæcal material. In these cases, when seen early enough, I have known all the signs of intussusception entirely disappear after being given *Opium* and without any operation at all.

There are strong indications for *Opium* in intestinal obstruction—cases of mechanical obstruction, such as strangulated hernia, volvulus, etc. Again there are the same group of symptoms—violent colicky pains with the sensation as though an attempt were being made to force something through a narrow passage which was completely blocked, the development of reverse peristalsis and, later, typical fæcal vomiting.

In all these cases, there is the same clinical picture: the feeling of acute abdominal distension, a sensation as though the abdomen were nearly bursting, and that if some flatus could be passed they would be better, but nothing is passed per rectum except, possibly, a little blood-stained mucus.

From the homœopathic prescribing point of view, there are several typical features which have to be present in order to individualise the *Opium* case. The first is the incessant nausea. The patients, as a rule, have no appetite at all, and reject any suggestion of food. There is an exception—in a certain number of cases of paralytic ileus there is a horrid, empty, sinking sensation which may be described as hunger, but from which eating brings no relief.

These patients complain of intense thirst and a persistently dry mouth which nothing will relieve. In cases of paralytic ileus with the patient vomiting pints of fluid, it is not surprising that he should be as dry as a bone. Also with this condition there is frequently a very dry, furred tongue. It may be simply a white coating to the tongue or, if the condition has progressed, a thick brownish-black coating. But it is the intense dryness of the tongue that is the outstanding feature.

Another pointer to *Opium* is that all these patients are worse after they have been asleep. You are often told that the patient was moderately comfortable and fell asleep, he slept for a period of twenty minutes or half an hour and then began to twitch a little—his arms twitched, his legs twitched—and finally he woke up complaining of very severe headache. Immediately on beginning to move, he felt violently sick and brought up pints of this bile-stained fluid. During these attacks, the abdomen becomes extremely sensitive to touch and to pressure.

Quite frequently, there is the history that these patients get very much worried at night, they tend to become delirious and have extreme night terrors, of horrible, terrifying visions.

In appearance, when at rest these patients tend to look horribly drawn and almost withered. With the acute attack of colic they flush up and may become actually cyanosed; they also tend to become sweaty, the skin feeling very hot and moist.

In the acute attacks of pain, the pupils become contracted. When the attack is over, there is an appearance of extreme exhaustion and the patient is hardly able to keep his eyes open. During the night terrors these patients sometimes have widely-open, staring eyes, but without the contracted pupils normally associated with *Opium*.

Complicating their thirst, these patients often complain of a spasmodic feeling in the œsophagus on swallowing; they may have actual difficulty in getting fluids down, and the attempt may make them sick.

I remember seeing one man with a paralytic ileus in whom this symptom was very marked. He was simply parched with thirst, his tongue was as dry as a parrot's; but if he took a few sips of water, up it came—followed immediately by the best part of a pint of green bilious vomit. He responded at once to a few doses of *Opium* and made an excellent recovery.

A striking point about the *Opium* pains is the manner in which the patients describe them, saying that they actually feel that they have an obstruction. The man I mentioned said he felt as if his stomach contracted and tried to force the contents through a narrow outlet which seemed to be blocked; the whole process was then reversed, the contents swished back into the other end of the stomach and came up his throat, he could not control it and the fluid simply poured out.

After he became convalescent, this patient had a recurrence of a similar sensation in his pyloric region. He described this as though there were a tight band narrowing his pylorus, and as though his food could not get through it, and he insisted on having another X-ray (which was negative) to see if he had not got adhesions tying down his duodenum and obstructing the passage. *Opium* entirely cleared up this symptom and he had no recurrence. This is the commonest description of *Opium* that will be given.

Another description of the discomfort of *Opium* is that there is a hard lump—almost like a stone—in the abdomen, which obstructs the passage of the intestinal contents.

The colic of *Opium* is every bit as violent as that of *Colocynth*: the patients have such intense pain that it feels as if their bowels were being cut to pieces. (That description may be met with in any obstructive condition.)

Occasionally there are indications for *Opium* in cases of organic—that is to say, carcinomatous—stricture of the bowel where there are definite obstructive symptoms and acute colicky pains, with a horrid obstructed sensation and the involuntary passage of small quantities of rather offensive diarrhœic stool.

One ordinarily associates the *Opium* picture with the hot-blooded, flushed, cyanotic, somewhat apoplectic patient. But in these abdominal cases, there is likely to be a sensation of heat and general congestion tending to be confined to the head and neck, very often with a cold, clammy sweat over the rest of the body, particularly the extremities.

It is obvious that though the sphere of action of *Opium* may be a little limited, it is a very important emergency drug. One should know it well for when called for it is of immense value.

ORNITHOGALUM

ALTHOUGH this drug has only been imperfectly proved, it is a very useful one. Our use of *Ornithogalum* is restricted entirely to pyloric ulcers and gastric or pyloric carcinomas.

There are certain characteristic symptoms which help one to prescribe it. Unless these are present the drug has very little effect. I have seen it prescribed in a haphazard way for pyloric carcinoma with no benefit at all, and I have seen it prescribed with very great benefit. On the one hand it was prescribed simply on the pathology of the case, and on the other it was prescribed on the pathology plus the distinguishing symptoms.

There are certain symptoms connected with this drug which are purely pathological. For instance, a feeling of extreme pressure, distension in the epigastrium described as a horrible feeling as if the whole upper abdomen or lower part of the chest were completely full up; very often a foul taste in the mouth, and severe constipation. On examination, you often find that the abdomen is definitely enlarged, frequently with obvious enlargement of the superficial veins, and a very much enlarged liver.

The individualising symptoms of *Ornithogalum* are several. There are very characteristic pains, described as a feeling as if an attempt were being made to force something through a narrow passage in the stomach, the pyloric region or the chest. These pains seem to spread all over the body: they spread right down into the hands, into the arms and through to the back, particularly just between the shoulders. The pains tend to be very much worse at night. They are slightly relieved by warm foods, and are aggravated by cold drinks.

In the early stages, where the lesion is pyloric, the patients are relieved by food. Unfortunately the indications for *Ornithogalum* in these early cases are apt to be missed, or the patients do not seek advice until this early stage is passed. So far as I know, there is no record of any definite food likes or dislikes.

There is a horrid feeling of restlessness—the patients say they cannot keep still—and this feeling is associated with a very unpleasant, creepy feeling in the legs. There is also a marked tendency in *Ornithogalum* cases towards the early development of œdema of the lower limbs.

They get another peculiar sensation, as if the stomach were full of water—just as if there were a loose bag of water which tended to drag to either side when they turned over. Mechanically, it is the kind of symptom you would expect from their pyloric obstruction and resultant dilated stomach. It is a very marked symptom in *Ornithogalum*, and is sometimes very useful.

These patients are always bringing up a quantity of offensive gas, but this does not appreciably relieve their feeling of distension.

With the sensation that something is being forced through in the pyloric region, the patients often complain that they feel as if they swell up into little hard lumps in various parts of the epigastrium or throughout the abdomen; and they very often feel as if, after a gurgle, this little lump begins to subside again.

Not infrequently they feel extremely chilly before the attacks of pain develop, or just as the pain is beginning to become acute.

Not unnaturally in this state, the patients are usually extremely depressed and may be actually suicidal. They have much the same restlessness as *Arsenicum*, but without the *Arsenicum* fear.

There are two further points. One is that *Ornithogalum* patients, with their carcinomatous lesion, tend to have a very clean red tongue with a coated base. The other is that, with their feeling of abdominal distension, they get a strange sensation of pressure throughout the whole body, which is described as feeling as if all their nerves were in a state of tension.

It is allied to the tingling, distressing sensation they get in their legs associated with œdema, but they get it in areas where there is no œdema at all; it is very much the feeling of fullness that they may get anywhere. As the condition progresses they get nausea and vomiting. The vomit will be typical of gastric or pyloric carcinoma, either mucus or mucus and blood.

One should look critically at the mode of administration of *Ornithogalum*. Those who have used it most are insistent that it should be given in unit doses of the tincture. In the majority of cases which I have seen treated by *Ornithogalum*, unit doses of the tincture have been employed. However, I have seen two cases of undoubted carcinoma which responded rather better to single doses of a 200 potency than any case that I have seen on unit doses of the tincture.

These two cases had very obvious *Ornithogalum* general symptoms as well as the local ones. The unit dose of the tincture has been so strongly recommended because the medicine has been given mainly on pathological grounds, without much attention being paid to the general symptoms; and *Ornithogalum* does seem to have a specific effect on pyloric growths.

Ornithogalum is a very useful drug and one which we cannot afford to forget. At worst, the most hopeless, inoperable cases can be made more comfortable under its action, even though it may not prove curative. But there are numerous records of its curative action and I have myself seen several cases make a complete recovery after its administration where the outlook appeared to be absolutely hopeless.

PETROLEUM

PETROLEUM is another of the drugs which are very much overlooked. We tend to prescribe it for skin eruptions and nothing else, but it has a very definite place in the treatment of digestive disturbances. The indications for *Petroleum* are very clear, and cases calling for it respond exceedingly well.

The *Petroleum* patient is the anæmic, rather undernourished, chronic dyspeptic woman; and there is the history that the skin is very dry and rough and always tends to crack in winter. These patients get deep chaps on their hands. They always have some catarrhal discharge of some kind somewhere. It may be a chronic nasal discharge, a chronic discharging ear or a chronic leucorrhœa. And always, no matter where the catarrh is, there is the same type of thick, yellowish-green discharge.

They are always rather tired people, and frequently complain of a bruised feeling all over. It is very much like the tired, bruised sensation of *Arnica*.

In spite of being rather underweight, *Petroleum* patients have a very good appetite and it may be extreme and go on to a state of constant gnawing hunger. In the attacks of acute gastritis, they are liable to get pain coming on immediately after food. But if they are feeling sickish the feeling of nausea is usually relieved by eating.

Associated with the nausea, they complain of a feeling of faintness or of coldness in the abdomen. It is worth noting that they are extremely sensitive to motion—to rail journeys, car journeys and, particularly, to sailing.

Petroleum is one of the outstanding sea-sickness remedies for cases in which the sensation of nausea is better from eating and is associated with a sinking feeling in the abdomen, and a feeling of general coldness or of coldness in the abdomen.

Petroleum people often complain of coldness in various spots: in the stomach, in the abdomen, between the scapulae, or it may be a cold sensation round the heart.

Associated with the tendency to sea-sickness, most *Petroleum* patients are very liable to attacks of giddiness produced by any motion—car riding, train travelling and sailing.

They get extreme itching of the surfaces and complain of itching and irritation of the eyes and ears. In the cold weather they get horribly itching chilblains. They have intense irritation wherever there is any skin eruption; the cracks of their hands become intensely irritable, and they get vesicular eruptions all round the edges of the scalp, behind the ears and, particularly, where there is any discharge.

All *Petroleum* eruptions tend to be extremely itchy. It is said that after scratching they develop a sensation of coldness in the itchy part, but I have never come across it.

Mentally, these patients are quite interesting. They are very often rather excitable and liable to get angry at trifles. But, when not excited, they tend to be mentally dull and a little confused; and their confusion may become quite extreme so that they lose their way when going about.

They may get quite muddled, with the sensation that there is somebody approaching them, somebody near when there is nobody about. They are especially apt to get muddled at night, with a feeling of general confusion and almost the sensation as if there were somebody else in the bed beside them; or they have a feeling that they are double.

As regards their temperature reactions, they are very much worse in the cold, very sensitive to weather changes and to thunder. In winter their skin tends to crack and bleed and become very sore, and yet the acute irritation of the skin eruptions is much worse when they are warm in bed.

If they are out in the cold air, walking against a cold wind, they tend to get a feeling of acute oppression in the chest—a feeling of tiredness, almost a shortness of breath.

The actual digestive conditions from which they suffer may be anything from gastritis to a gastric ulcer, and they are liable to attacks of what one can only describe as chronic colitis.

In their stomach attacks they are liable to develop pretty acute gastric pain which tends to spread up into the chest, and is accompanied by nausea which is definitely relieved by eating.

In their colitis they get fairly violent attacks of colic—exactly the type described under *Colocynth.*—which doubles them up and is rather better for firm pressure. The whole colon is tender to pressure.

There is exceedingly violent, offensive diarrhœa, and the patients may be quite incontinent. The stool usually contains a quantity of mucus, is very often greenish in colour and may contain blood. The diarrhœa is liable to be very much worse during the day and better during the night.

Associated with colitis, *Petroleum* patients are liable to develop an acute catarrh of the bladder. Apart from the ordinary symptoms of a bladder catarrh, the *Petroleum* patients' bladder trouble is often accompanied by intense irritation in the back part of the urethra, and this gives rise to acute discomfort in bed.

As regards likes and dislikes, there is a definite aversion to meat, fats and to most hot foods. The patients are somewhat finicky in their food desires: rather than having any definite specific cravings they want the appetite tickled by something pleasant or unusual.

The diarrhœa is very much aggravated by any vegetables, particularly coarse ones, such as cabbage.

One other *Petroleum* characteristic: these chronic dyspeptics with their general anæmia and loss of weight, often complain that their hair is falling out in handfuls.

PHOSPHORICUM ACIDUM

PHOSPHORIC ACID provides the classical picture of the painless, almost incontinent, watery, non-odorous diarrhœa. But the drug has a field of usefulness far greater than that, and it is one of the most useful drugs we have for the acid dyspepsia of the late adolescent. The kind of case is that of the child who is working for scholarship examinations and getting over-tired and whose digestion is beginning to give out.

This idea of the overstressed adolescent gives you the key to the whole picture; you get the same kind of condition at any age in anyone who has been under stress—particularly mental stress over a length of time—and who is beginning to break down. There may be indications for *Phosphoric acid* in more acute cases, such as bad shock, but it is much more commonly indicated after a period of prolonged stress.

The mental picture is that of those who are just dead tired. They feel generally indefinite, do not want to talk, cannot concentrate, their thoughts wander away from the subject. Any mental effort is liable to produce an acute headache with a sensation of extreme pressure on the top of the head. On any effort at all these patients are liable to feel giddy.

It is not an acute giddiness but a feeling of general instability, and patients quite frequently describe it as a feeling as if their feet were coming up off the ground and they would fall. Where you get indications for *Phosphoric acid* in acute illness—for example, in typhoid fever—this sensation is described as a feeling as if they were floating off the bed; but you get a minor degree of the same kind of thing even when the patients are going about.

One outstanding characteristic about *Phosphoric acid* patients is the astonishing relief they get from even quite a short sleep. You often see them just dead beat—you can hardly get a word out of them—then they have a short sleep (fifteen or twenty minutes) and wake up entirely different beings, their headache has gone and they are quite bright and cheery.

However, any little exertion, mental or physical, seems to use them up again and they slip back to the same state: their headache returns and they are just useless. With such a picture, the digestive disturbance most commonly met with is the complete failure of digestion. The digestion is slow, and the patients feel distended and uncomfortable after a meal. They may feel sick, and may vomit a quantity of sour, undigested food some hours after a meal.

Notably associated with the distension—often described as pressure—there is a general sensation of tightness or pressure. They may get it in the head or in the eyes, if they are using them much. They get exactly the same feeling of tightness in the chest on exertion and have generalised rheumatic pains with the same kind of feeling of pressure in the joints and they often complain of pressing pains in the soles of the feet.

Gastric discomfort is very much relieved by warm food or warm drinks. This is the outstanding differentiating point between *Phosphoric acid* and *Phosphorus*.

Another symptom in *Phosphoric acid* digestive disturbances is an excessive amount of flatulence. These tired-out patients very often complain of constant rumbling or gurgling in the abdomen.

There is a strange hyperæsthesia in these apparently sluggish patients: they are very sensitive to music, very easily startled and often peculiarly sensitive to odours.

Temperature reactions are a little contradictory. The patients are chilly, sensitive to cold, particularly sensitive to wind, very sensitive to snow atmospheres; and yet, in a hot room they are upset, their headaches are made worse and their mental sluggishness is increased. They are fresher and their headaches are better in the open air, provided it is still.

It is characteristic that they appear to get the most acute gastric discomfort about half an hour after a meal. At that time there is a tendency for the food simply to regurgitate into the throat, and this regurgitation may be accompanied by cramping pains in the stomach.

They are upset by any acid foods, by fresh fruit, cold drinks, or by any over-rich food. Frequently, *Phosphoric acid* patients are rather thirsty. They tend to have a definite polyuria with a very pale, milky kind of urine and, when that is present, they complain of a very dry mouth and intense thirst.

Another odd characteristic of *Phosphoric acid* patients is their liability to develop styes. The styes particularly affect the upper lids

In adolescents with students' headaches, there may be a tendency for the right pupil to be rather larger than the left. This may be slight or it may be marked, and it is particularly noticeable during a headache.

There is sometimes a complaint of a tendency to bite the tongue during sleep. This is commonly associated with acute gastric disturbances.

In adolescents the picture is not unlike that of *Pulsatilla*, but it has its own characteristics which should make it clear. In adults the picture is much more clear and individual, and the selection is correspondingly easier.

PHOSPHORUS

THE greatest use for *Phosphorus* is in acute gastric ulcers. There may be indications for it in cases of jaundice—acute jaundice with congestion of the liver—and there may also be indications in acute diarrhœas; but the commonest digestive condition in which it is required is the acute gastric ulcer.

The condition is a very acute one, with acute burning pain in the stomach. It is frequently accompanied by a very bitter or sour taste in the mouth; and there is often a complaint that the food tastes unnatural, either salty or sweetish. With the bitter taste, patients often complain of acute salivation and of the mouth generally feeling sore and hot.

In spite of the burning pains in the stomach, there is a horrible faint, hungry sensation which returns again quite soon after a meal. There is always great thirst and a constant desire for cold fluids. The cold things which are taken relieve the burning in the stomach for a time—anything up to half an hour.

In characteristic *Phosphorus* vomiting, mouthfuls of material are eructated and this goes on persistently until the stomach has been emptied. This is much the most common story; but there may be a feeling of constant nausea with a sense of distension and then a sudden violent vomit of a quantity of bright blood. This is liable to be followed by recurring attacks of nausea, burning pain and a tendency to bring up quantities of coffee-ground or black vomit.

As far as the desire for food and drink is concerned, in acute conditions all that is wanted is sips of cold water or some cold juicy fluid. In the less acute stage the desire is for spicy or tasty things—salt food or generally refreshing food. There is also a liking for sour things and, often, for stimulating wines. There is a marked aversion to sweets, boiled milk puddings and, often to meat, tea and coffee. Tea very often definitely aggravates the complaints.

Such is the ordinary stomach condition. You may be dealing with an acute gastritis with a general oozing from the mucous membrane, with an acute gastric ulcer or with a gastric carcinoma.

In general make-up, there is the typical *Phosphorus* appearance—the rather delicate, somewhat emaciated, tired and yet excitable, irritable, sensitive patient. These patients very much dislike being alone; are responsive to sympathy and much soothed by being stroked. They are very sensitive to thunder and to noise; liable to be a bit apprehensive, particularly in the dark; worse from any excitement, which is likely to produce a sensation of general pulsation, and sensitive to odours and to music. As a rule they are rather pale, but under any stress they flush up very easily. They are a little apt to become unduly depressed, just dejected and miserable.

As they become weaker, these patients rapidly develop extreme tremor of the hands and become very shaky—this is very noticeable on any excitement.

They are definitely chilly patients, sensitive to cold and to strong winds. They get a feeling of oppression, tightness, embarrassment of breathing on any attempt to walk against a wind.

With the disturbances of the lower digestive tract, you have to deal with chronic enteritis; and there are sometimes indications for *Phosphorus* in cases of chronic pancreatitis or in acute jaundice. In any of these conditions the patient's complaint is very similar. There is a feeling as if the whole abdomen were sensitive, painful, tender, and as if the abdominal contents were hanging down. This is accompanied by a good deal of rumbling and gurgling in the abdomen. Very often the gurgle starts in the stomach, seems to run right down through the alimentary tract and is followed by an involuntary stool.

The patients get a good deal of flatulence and colic and are liable to very troublesome attacks of diarrhœa. The stool is usually rather offensive, with a considerable amount of colic before the bowels act, and there is liable to be very violent tenesmus afterwards. Not infrequently after these attacks of diarrhœa, there is a tendency to prolapse with the violent tenesmus, which is extremely painful.

In more chronic conditions, *Phosphorus* patients often complain of a horrible, empty, sinking sensation about 11 a.m.

As may be expected with jaundice or pancreatitis, there is liable to be a bileless stool—quite white, watery and offensive.

In attacks of diarrhœa, they frequently have acute palpitations following stool. In any of their disturbances, they complain bitterly of intense coldness of the extremities, particularly the legs and feet.

PHYTOLACCA

THE main uses one finds for *Phytolacca* are in very severe gastric ulcers, gastric carcinomas and, occasionally, rectal carcinomas.

It is a little difficult to give a clear picture of *Phytolacca* patients, but in most cases they are very depressed, gloomy and rather indifferent. In addition to their local symptoms they always feel very tired and often complain of generalised bruised pains, a sort of aching pain all over. They are also very liable to severe bone pains which are particularly troublesome in bed at night.

With rectal carcinomas, they are particularly liable to get a most troublesome backache, a throbbing type of pain in the lumbar or sacral region. This also tends to be much worse at night and is particularly bad in a warm bed.

The patients are sensitive to cold; they feel chilly, are very sensitive to damp and to cold rooms. And yet, in most of their complaints they have an aggravation from getting overheated in bed at night.

The appearance of the tongue is a little suggestive. As a rule it has a very coated base—a yellowish, dry base—and with a very red tip. Usually the patients have been liable to attacks of sore throat, they have rather large tonsils, and there is often a bluish appearance of the back of the throat and of the pillars of the fauces. They complain of a raw, rough sensation in the throat, and of severe stiffness in the neck as if the muscles at the sides of the neck were rigid.

In their gastric disturbances, the main complaint is of pain in the pyloric region. After food they get a feeling as if the whole stomach were contracting—they express it as feeling as if the stomach were being pinched together—and they tell you that soon after a meal they feel a sinking, hungry sensation and then begin to get the pyloric pain, become sick and vomit. The vomit may be variable but—certainly with carcinoma—it usually consists of a quantity of blood-stained slimy mucus.

In carcinoma cases, there is usually a good deal of pain in the region of the liver. The liver is sensitive to pressure, and the pain is very much worse when the patient is turned over on to the right side.

As a rule, the gastric discomfort is relieved by hot drinks.

In rectal carcinoma, there are one or two suggestive symptoms. The patients complain of a good deal of generalised abdominal discomfort, a feeling of rumbling in the abdomen and an almost constant urging to stool. With this urging, they pass only a little blood-stained mucus, or else they pass little shreddy discharges which look almost like the lining of the mucous membrane and are stained with blood. With this rectal condition, they get very acute neuralgic pain in the rectum and anus. This pain tends to spread forward into the perineum.

These are the main points about *Phytolacca*. If the patients have always been liable to get enlarged inflamed glands—particularly of the glands of the neck—or they have been liable to attacks of recurring mastitis, or acute sensitiveness and swelling of the mammae at the menstrual periods—these are extra indications for *Phytolacca* in the more acute pyloric ulcers.

The range of *Phytolacca* is rather limited, but it does fill a definite gap where one is dealing with these malignant conditions which are very often difficult to fit with a drug.

PLUMBUM

IT is very difficult to give a coherent story of the uses of *Plumbum* because it seems to fit such different conditions.

Plumbum is occasionally indicated in infancy. The child is wasted and shrivelled-looking, with a very large abdomen and obstinate constipation, and a history of violent attacks of abdominal colic which make him double up. The infant has a very offensive odour, sweaty skin, cold hands and feet, a very coated tongue and, in addition to the abdominal colic, is liable to attacks of cramp or generalised spasms. He has no appetite at all, and refuses any food or drink.

There is another *Plumbum* type at the other end of life: a patient who has had a cerebral hæmorrhage, a flaccid paralysis of one or other side and is suffering from the most obstinate constipation—particularly if the constipation is associated with abdominal colic. In these cases, there is the slow mentality of the post-apoplectic, a general mild depression and faulty memory.

Instead of the general abdominal distension of the infant, there is much more likely to be a somewhat retracted abdomen; and the complaint of feeling as if the abdomen were being pulled in. They get sudden attacks of violent colic, in which the pains are rather better from pressure and eructation of wind.

It is not only at the two extremes of life that one gets indications for *Plumbum*. There may be indications for *Plumbum* in the chlorosis of late adolescence where it is associated with obstinate constipation, a generalised mild anæmia, a very sallow, somewhat greasy skin and complete loss of appetite.

There will be, in addition, the peculiar *Plumbum* mental picture of sluggish mentality, with poor memory, frightfully slow mental reaction and—in spite of the general mental sluggishness—a history that the patients find difficulty in sleeping.

In these cases, the patients may suffer from a somewhat chronic gastric catarrh. There is a feeling of nausea, a complaint that everything seems to turn sour; and the vomiting of quantities of sour material. In spite of everything turning sour, they sometimes complain of a very troublesome sweetish taste in the mouth. They are liable to violent attacks of hiccough. Frequently they have a very dry, red, glazed-looking tongue.

These cases suffer from obstinate constipation, often accompanied by an acute spasm about the anus on any attempt at defacation and a feeling as if the anus were being pulled right up into the rectum. Associated with the constipation, they often complain of very severe pain in the cecal region. They are liable to suffer from acute headaches with the constipation; and complain that the effort to get the bowels to act is so extreme that they are completely exhausted by it.

With the constipation and chlorosis, these patients very frequently suffer from crops of boils.

Plumbum chlorotic adolescents are always neurasthenics and they are very liable to sham all sorts of illnesses which they have not got, particularly ailments associated with some kind of paretic symptoms. They say they feel almost paralysed, or they cannot use an arm or a leg—and they sham beautifully until they think there is no one watching them.

These neurotic patients often give a history of attacks of difficulty in swallowing, as if there were a spasm of the œsophagus which made them choke.

These patients are very often troubled with cold, sweaty, very offensive feet. They complain that the skin of the feet, particularly between the toes, is almost as if it had been steeped in water and looks half macerated.

Plumbum patients are intensely chilly, particularly sensitive to damp and upset by any exertion. They have one very peculiar symptom: *the more they walk in the open air, the colder their legs and feet become.* It is a symptom I have come across several times in these abdominal neurasthenics.

There are two other conditions which give indications for *Plumbum*. One is acute jaundice, in which there is a very dry, shrivelled appearance with the typical jaundiced skin; very constant, very marked, acute nausea and persistent vomiting. There is acute constipation and pretty acute pain in the liver which is very tender, tender to pressure; and the pain extends right through to the back, sometimes right over to the left side. The vomit is a green, bilious, mucous vomit.

These cases of jaundice have a heavily coated tongue, and there is liable to be generalised muscular cramps. For *Plumbum* to be indicated, there must also be the *Plumbum* mentality, the general sluggishness, depression and complete loathing of food or drink of any kind.

The other condition which may give indications for *Plumbum* is intestinal obstruction. As you would expect in these cases, the patients get most violent abdominal colic, a feeling as if everything were churning up and an acute spasm were trying to force it past the obstruction.

But the characteristic *Plumbum* sensation is a feeling as if everything were being drawn backwards up against the posterior abdominal wall, or a feeling as if there were acute retraction of the umbilicus, as if it were being tugged in.

There is complete obstruction—no action of the bowel at all—extreme nausea, the vomit first consisting of food—ordinary gastric contents—then becoming sour, bilious and, finally, fæcal. All this is accompanied by very persistent hiccough, extreme sensitiveness of the abdomen to pressure—the slightest contact with the abdominal wall being painful—general cold, offensive sweat and typical loathing of anything taken by mouth.

Plumbum may be indicated in intestinal obstruction at any age. I have seen it indicated in children with strangulated hernia, in intussusception in infants and in intestinal obstruction from intestinal carcinoma.

I remember one patient who had a carcinoma at the splenic flexure; she had typical indications for *Plumbum*, which stopped her spasms for months on end. She had no morphia at all, though before having *Plumbum* she had been having pretty heavy doses of morphia without any benefit—it was merely making her sick.

The strange thing was that at the post mortem she was found to have an almost complete obstruction even though, after *Plumbum* she had started to pass some fæcal material: how it got through was a mystery but the obstruction was up in her splenic flexure where the contents are still pretty liquid.

With these inoperable conditions one can give enormous relief with homœopathy by prescribing accurately on their symptoms. A very small dose of morphia will keep the patients quite comfortable if they are having homœopathic treatment whereas, without it, they would be requiring half grains of morphia four hourly.

I remember a child in the children's ward whom everyone believed had an intussusception. While he was waiting for the operation and to get him into a fit state, as he was very shocked, he was given three doses of *Plumbum*, and all his symptoms disappeared. He had had all the symptoms of intussusception and yet, after *Plumbum*, they simply disappeared. It may be that the *Plumbum*, by relieving the spasm, allowed the intussusception to correct itself.

The boy was about two years old, and had been ill for three days. He was in a very collapsed condition, and was really only left to recover sufficiently to be fit for operation—instead of which he recovered altogether.

PODOPHYLLUM

THE ordinary conception of *Podophyllum* as a drug for summer diarrhœa is far too restricted. Although it is immensely useful in summer diarrhœa, it has a sphere of action very much greater than that.

The type of summer diarrhœa in children in which *Podophyllum* is so very useful is that in which there is the most profuse, very offensive, watery diarrhœa, accompanied by the passage of a quantity of very offensive flatus, associated with acute abdominal colic and with signs of very acute prostration.

It is usually associated, in these summer diarrhœas, with signs of a certain amount of meningeal irritation, sometimes amounting to no more than a constant rolling of the head from side to side, though there may be actual retraction of the neck. Very commonly, this is associated with a constant chewing motion of the maw, there may be actual grinding of the teeth if the child is a little older; and, not infrequently, there is a definite squint. It is not a true meningitis: on lumbar puncture there may be slightly increased pressure, but no abnormal cerebro-spinal fluid.

This type of summer diarrhœa does respond very well to *Podophyllum*, but it is only a very small part of the story. You get indications for *Podophyllum* in all sorts of gastro-intestinal catarrhs, very often with an extension up the bile ducts and a definite cholecystitis. Occasionally there may be indications for it in gall-stones, although that is not so common.

The patients mainly complain of constant discomfort after any food, and feel as if they were stuffed full. With this feeling, they say that they cannot digest anything, everything seems to turn sour. Associated with the spoiled sensation in the stomach they have frequent attacks of acute salivation and belch up a quantity of sour wind. They often have a burning sensation in the throat and a burning tongue, accompanied by intense thirst and a desire for cold drinks.

In all digestive disturbances, these patients get a very thickly coated tongue, particularly at the root. The tongue as a whole is often somewhat soft, flabby and pale, with a very thick yellow coating at the base.

The vomit may be anything from sourish fluid to definite bile, depending on the extension of the catarrh—whether it is merely gastric or has spread down into the duodenum or involves the liver. When the liver is involved, they usually have pretty extreme nausea and aversion to every kind of food—they simply cannot bear the sight of it.

They get a good deal of pain in the liver, which is very much worse from pressure, the pain extends right through to the back and is somewhat relieved by gentle stroking, particularly stroking from behind forwards in the region of the liver. These somewhat jaundiced patients often sit up in bed, just stroking the liver, trying to shift something. They find some relief from it, although the subcostal region will be very sensitive to pressure.

In the catarrhal attacks, the patients tend to be very depressed, almost melancholy; and, if the pain is troublesome, they may become very fidgety and restless. In acute attacks, they frequently run a temperature, and may then have profuse night sweats.

There is a more chronic condition with a history of the patients having "liver upsets" as they call them—digestive upsets with a feeling of fullness in the upper abdomen and a general dragging sensation in the lower abdomen. With an attack of diarrhœa, they get a severe dragged sensation in the abdomen and feel extremely faint.

Before the bowels act, there is a sensation of fullness in the rectum, with a good deal of generalised abdominal rumbling and gurgling. After the bowels have moved, they have a feeling as if the rectum would prolapse, an increase of the dragging sensation and a horrible feeling of faintness.

In spite of their distress, they often say they prefer to have an attack of diarrhœa because if they become at all constipated they are liable to suffer from very severe occipital headaches. It is a sort of bilious, sick headache which these people describe, with a loathing for all food, general depression and a disinclination to do anything.

Typical *Podophyllum* patients are sensitive to cold. Their attacks of colic are relieved by externally applied warmth. Their attacks of diarrhœa are likely to be precipitated by any acid fruit, sometimes by milk, and very often by vegetables—particularly the coarser vegetables of the cabbage type.

Not infrequently these attacks of diarrhœa occur in the early hours of the morning, between 2 and 5 o'clock. The diarrhœa is very urgent and, if the call is not attended to at once, there is liable to be incontinence.

Occasionally, *Podophyllum* is indicated for women who suffer from recurring attacks of diarrhœa at their periods. Where the patient has made rather a slow recovery after a confinement and has a sensation of abdominal drag all the time.

She probably has a bulky uterus, and at the period the uterus feels very heavy; she may even have the sensation of a prolapse developing. This, associated with recurring attacks of diarrhœa at the periods, will very often be controlled by *Podophyllum* which materially improves the pelvic condition.

One other condition in which *Podophyllum* can be very helpful is the constant urging to stool accompanying rectal carcinoma. There is a history of alternating attacks of diarrhœa and constipation, of pretty violent tenesmus at stool with difficulty in passing stool; of a feeling as if the rectum were being forced out and a prolapse were developing, and of violent straining to pass a little offensive blood and mucus.

This condition is frequently controlled by *Podophyllum*. Several rectal carcinomas have very materially diminished under the action of *Podophyllum*; it not only controls the discomfort but seems actually to control the growth.

One old man had an extensive, inoperable carcinoma. He had known that he had it for about eighteen months before I saw him His story was that he got recurring attacks of diarrhœa and constipation, and when he was developing an attack of diarrhœa he used to get awful rumbling and gurgling in his abdomen and then a sudden urge to stool, which he could hardly control. The stools were very offensive; he nearly collapsed after each action and often had pretty violent and painful tenesmus.

He went on for two to two and a half years on occasional doses of *Podophyllum*. He went slowly downhill (incidentally, he died from an intercurrent pneumonia which he developed while he was in the country) but from the time of my first seeing him, his carcinoma certainly diminished in size. When I first saw him, I could not insert the tip of my finger into the annular stricture: when I last saw him, about two and a half years later, I could pass my forefinger through quite comfortably. And, from being incontinent, he had regained complete control.

He died of an intercurrent disease, and whether he would have recovered from his carcinoma had he survived, I do not know; but the amount of relief he got from *Podophyllum* was simply astonishing.

PSORINUM

WE tend to associate *Psorinum* with the patient who is inordinately hungry, but there is another picture which fits in with *Psorinum* in purely digestive disturbances: the patient who is making a very slow convalescence from an acute illness, who has no appetite at all and in whom all digestion seems to have ceased. Everything seems to turn sour in the stomach and there is a great deal of sour, or very offensive, eructation.

It is the kind of patient who is very difficult to fit with a medicine because individualising symptoms on which to prescribe are so lacking—the patient is just dead tired, there seems to be no reaction at all, and he drags along without picking up. Often there is an extreme empty feeling in the abdomen, but with a complete loathing of food.

These patients are nearly always constipated, and their constipation is rather suggestive. It consists of a complete inability to evacuate the rectum although the stool is perfectly soft. What stool is passed is always foully offensive, and is often accompanied by very offensive flatus. They get a good deal of flatulence, and complain that the flatus, as well as being offensive, is very hot and burning when it is passed.

They also complain of nausea, starting about 10 a.m., accompanied by a very sweetish, unpleasant regurgitation of fluid. These convalescents develop an acute intolerance of tobacco; any attempt at smoking is liable to bring on the most violent hiccough.

They are just dead beat: their main desire is to be left alone, to be allowed to lie down and not exert themselves in any way. Any exertion is liable to cause violent perspiration which tends to be very offensive; and they not infrequently suffer from offensive night sweats.

They suffer from extreme giddiness on exertion in the open air, are very chilly—especially about the head and neck—and mostly have a very unhealthy mouth and, often, extensive pyorrhœa.

Psorinum patients are always very depressed, they feel quite hopeless, they are never going to get better; and not infrequently complain that, owing to their illness, their business is going downhill and they are going to be ruined.

They are very sensitive to any change of temperature and to thunderstorms. They simply cannot bear any draught of air. They often tell you that they simply cannot breathe in cold air.

Frequently these patients complain of intensely irritant eruptions on the skin. But, apart from eruptions, they get intense itching which is very troublesome at night in bed when they get warm, and is very much aggravated by any woollen clothing or by bathing.

When they are perspiring, they often have a very greasy-looking appearance of the face; though the skin of the legs, arms and hands may be very dry, harsh and rough, liable to crack and always giving a very dirty appearance.

Occasionally, there are indications for *Psorinum* in acute infantile diarrhœas. The child is very unhealthy-looking, with a rough, dirty-looking, coarse skin which is liable to crack and become sore in cold weather. Frequently, the child has blepharitis, red, unhealthy-looking eyes and a chronic nasal discharge. There is a history of steady loss of weight, although the appetite is good, sometimes even inordinate. And, he has gone down with a very violent attack of diarrhœa.

The youngsters seem to be quite incapable of sleeping, they are fretful and irritable all the time and cannot rest. There is constant irritation in the abdomen, with rumbling and gurgling; and the most violent, stinking, brown, watery diarrhœa. The children are usually incontinent.

If you get a history that the diarrhœa started as the result of a chill, it not infrequently responds to *Psorinum*.

There is one thing, apart from the general dirty appearance, that always makes me think of *Psorinum* for these children: they often have a peculiar fuzzy growth of fine hair on the face.

It is very difficult to repertorise a drug for the ill-defined malaise and poor reaction of the unsatisfactory convalescent; and a knowledge of the symptom picture of *Psorinum* will often prove immensely useful in such cases.

PTELIA

PTELIA is a drug which is very useful in the chronic dyspeptic.

You find indications for it in the weak, languid, tired-out dyspeptic. The patients are always rather dull and somewhat muddle-headed. Under stimulation they can become quite lively and cheerful, but whenever the stimulus goes, they relapse into the same dull, rather muddled, depressed state.

They complain of a constant digestive discomfort. Usually described as a feeling of a lump in the stomach or in the upper abdomen, but in spite of this, there is very often a sensation of hunger. One of the most marked characteristics is that the dullness and sluggishness is very much ameliorated after food—and, after a meal, they are very often quite lively and cheery. In spite of this mental uplift after a meal, there is often an increase of the abdominal fullness and heaviness.

They often complain that they are very clumsy in their movements. Their fingers feel numb, swollen and stiff, and it is very difficult for them to do any fine work at all.

These patients are sensitive to a stuffy atmosphere, and are better in cool air. They are liable to be much more heavy and muddle-headed in the mornings and, usually, after sleep at any time. And they wake up with a very dirty, unpleasant mouth.

Ptelia patients have a strong aversion to fats of any kind or any rich food, which aggravates their condition, and often they are definitely upset by anything in the nature of a milky pudding, and they have a very marked aversion to meat. With their dirty mouth, they very often have a desire for acids—sour things with a bit of a sting about them that taste clean. Not uncommonly, their major abdominal discomfort comes on about an hour after a meal.

Sometimes there is a certain amount of enlargement and tenderness of the liver, associated with a dull, generalised, bilious headache. The liver is uncomfortable, it may be a little tender when they are lying on the right side; and very often there is a sensation of weight and dragging in the liver region when the patient turns over to the left.

Some of the cases that get *Sepia* owing to their dull, depressed, negative sort of outlook would be better with *Ptelia*; and, where there is a marked aversion to meat, it is always worthwhile considering *Ptelia* as a possibility.

PULSATILLA

PULSATILLA is one of the typical flatulent dyspeptics. The patients get a feeling of general abdominal distension, they suffer from flatulence and very often have complete loss of appetite. They complain of a very dry mouth, sometimes with a bitter taste, and yet there is a complete absence of thirst.

They often say that they can taste their food hours after it is eaten —it seems not to digest at all—and when eating it feels as if the food stuck in the throat. This regurgitation, or taste, of food comes on about an hour or an hour and a half after a meal, and patients frequently say the food comes about halfway up the throat, sticks there and then goes back again.

In attacks of nausea and vomiting, they often complain of feeling horribly chilly. And yet, in any warm atmosphere, they get flushed and develop an acute sweat about the face and, in spite of their general chilliness, their nausea is made very much worse.

The eructation of *Pulsatilla*, when not tasting of food, is very often bitter or sour, and sometimes definitely fatty. The patients complain of the mouth feeling horribly slimy in the morning; and they suffer from acute heartburn, very often with a raw, scraped sensation in the throat and a burning sensation in the stomach. The burning sensation is very much aggravated by taking any warm food, and is temporarily relieved by cold fluids or cold food.

They tell you that when they are feeling most bloated, full up, they very often get relief from walking about gently in the open air. This also seems to relieve their sense of nausea.

These digestive upsets are always made worse by any rich food, particularly by any fat; and they are liable to get digestive upsets if they have been living too well. They not infrequently get a digestive upset—either in the way of abdominal cramp, sickness or diarrhœa—from taking very cold food, such as ice cream, particularly if they are overheated.

They develop a definite aversion to any fatty or greasy food; to meat, milk, bread, pastry and port. And they very often have the oddest desires for all sorts of indigestible foods with a definite taste; for sour foods, highly-seasoned things or very juicy fruits.

They often have a longing for cakes and pastry, in spite of being upset by them. Although they have no thirst, they often have an acute craving for acid fluids. This tends to be particularly marked in association with the unpleasant slimy condition of the mouth in the morning.

The condition from which they are most likely to suffer is a definite gastric or gastro-intestinal catarrh. Occasionally with the intestinal catarrh, they get a mild attack of jaundice and attacks of acute diarrhœa. There is acute abdominal colic, which tends to centre about the umbilicus, and is associated with intense chilliness and a sensation of nausea.

Sometimes they actually vomit, but more commonly they get a very violent diarrhœa with a burning sensation in the bowel and the passage of a quantity of mucus in the stool. The stools are very loose and watery, the diarrhœa tends to be much worse at night, and it is always accompanied by a good deal of flatus. In colour, the stools tend to be greenish, but the mucous character is the constant factor. In appearance, the stools vary very much from one action to another.

These attacks are liable to be brought on from exposure to cold, from iced food or drinks, from too much fruit.

When the catarrh extends to the liver, these patients complain of a good deal of pain—heavy dragging pain—in the region of the liver; and the pain extends right through to the back, between the shoulders. There may be a mild degree of jaundice, in which case there is usually a heavily furred, white tongue.

With liver attacks, *Pulsatilla* patients often complain of acute giddiness on first rising.

With the digestive upsets, you have, of course, the *Pulsatilla* make-up—general sensitiveness to a stuffy atmosphere, intolerance of heat, generally mild depression, slight nervousness of being left alone, a tendency to get worse in the latter part of the day (as evening comes on, the patient may become rather terrified), wanting to have somebody about, and craving for sympathy.

You get indications for *Pulsatilla* with alternation of gouty pains—particularly, gouty attacks which seem to wander from one joint to another—with digestive upsets. That is to say, when the digestion is fairly good, the gout returns, and when the gouty pains are better their digestion is worse.

The gouty pains are rather better from moving about gently, much worse from heat, and wander from joint to joint. These, alternating with digestive upsets of the above character, quite frequently respond to *Pulsatilla*. The tendency is to give *Kali bic.* to most of them but very often *Pulsatilla* would be better.

In *Pulsatilla* you will come across cases of constipation which exhibit all the local symptoms which one associates with *Nux vom.*—the ineffectual urging to stool with the feeling that they never get properly cleared. When these symptoms occur in a warm-blooded, gentle, yielding, *Pulsatilla* type of patient, you will fail entirely to get a response from *Nux vom.*; but, they will respond beautifully to *Pulsatilla*.

RAPHANUS

THE post-operative cases in which *Raphanus* is indicated are those in which there are signs suggesting intestinal obstruction, where there is a good deal of irregularly distributed abdominal distension, pockets of wind which the patient cannot move—they cannot get it up or pass it down.

There are very violent, twisting pains in the abdomen, sometimes in one part, sometimes in another, the position seeming to depend on where the flatus has stuck. It is usually associated with a good deal of nausea, and with a peculiar kind of drawing pain from the lower end of the sternum down into the umbilical region.

Always, there is marked thirst, but the spasms of pain are very much aggravated by drinking. Sometimes the patients complain of a good deal of burning discomfort in the epigastrium and of very small, scalding eructations.

Apart from the attacks of acute pain, there is a severe feeling of tightness in the abdomen. Some patients have described this as being almost as if they had an iron band right round the waist.

One peculiar symptom—they very often complain of icy cold knees.

In contrast to the state of acute distress, these patients have a peculiar mental attitude which can best be described as a feeling that they are finished and their number is up—and almost an acceptance of this. This attitude is in striking contrast to the state of acute terror which the thought of impending death produces in an *Arsenicum* patient suffering from a similar condition.

In post-operative cases of this kind, with patchy areas of distension, *Raphanus* is often much more useful than *Carbo veg.* or *Arsenicum*. In bad cases, it is certainly more useful than *Lycopodium*.

RHUS TOXICODENDRON

THERE are quite a number of conditions in which one finds indications for *Rhus tox.*, and the majority of them are very acute.

You may get indications for *Rhus tox.* in acute inflammatory disturbances of the œsophagus, usually the result of taking some scalding fluid or something of that sort. The outstanding characteristic is the intense pain. There is almost complete inability to swallow and any attempt to do so produces most violent, scalding pain all down the œsophagus.

This is associated with a very dry mouth and throat and the most violent thirst, with a desire for very cold drinks. Taking any cold fluid, however, produces a sensation of general chilliness.

Further indications for *Rhus tox.* may be found in a very acute gastritis with acute nausea and fairly violent vomit. There will be a history that the acute attack of gastritis has been brought on by taking very cold fluids, ice-cream or iced drinks in very hot weather—it is the result of a sudden chill.

Again there is the intense dryness of the mouth, with very violent thirst and the desire for cold drinks. Sometimes, there is desire for cold milk, which seems to comfort the stomach. On occasion in these attacks of acute gastritis, the *Rhus tox.* patients complain of a feeling of intense hunger, though they get sudden attacks of vomiting after taking any food.

There is another group of conditions in which one gets definite indications for *Rhus tox.*: acute inflammatory conditions in the abdomen. The commonest of these are acute appendicitis and acute generalised peritonitis. Acute dysentery is also common.

In the acute inflammatory abdominal condition, the abdomen is extremely sensitive to touch, the pains are pretty violent, and you will find the patients lying with the legs drawn up in order to relieve abdominal pressure. Most of the acute inflammatory conditions in the abdomen tend to be on the right side.

Not infrequently, you get indications for *Rhus tox.* in an appendicitis which is associated with a good deal of liver disturbance, either a cholecystitis or just a general congested liver with a degree of jaundice. In a typical *Rhus tox.* case of dysentery, there is the most violent tenesmus before and after stool, with acute abdominal colicky pains and the passage of bloody mucous stools.

You will occasionally see indications for *Rhus tox.* in typhoid. There are two stages at which this may occur. First, when the patients are having very violent, copious, watery stools, associated with a degree of tenesmus. Second, where there is complete incontinence—here, you are even more likely to observe *Rhus tox.* indications.

In both cases, the stools are much more frequent at night and much less frequent during the day. It is interesting to note that although one ordinarily associates *Rhus tox.* with bowel upsets which are accompanied by violent tenesmus and extreme straining at stool, in typhoid indications for *Rhus tox.* are much more likely to show themselves accompanied by complete incontinence.

In order to clinch a *Rhus tox.* diagnosis, there must be the general *Rhus tox.* modalities. The patients are always extremely tired. They are very despondent, and may be actually weepy. There is always a fairly marked anxious mental restlessness, and the patients may feel that they really want to die.

They nearly always complain of a feeling of general chilliness, and their discomforts are relieved by external warmth. In all their conditions, they complain of a degree of general stiffness, particularly after they have been still for a little time.

In all these painful conditions, they are restless, constantly on the move and find it impossible to keep still. This is one of the diagnostic points about the *Rhus tox.* appendicitis. Accompanying a somewhat distended right side of the abdomen, rigid muscles, acute tenderness to touch and relief from hot applications, the *Rhus tox.* patient is restless, constantly moving a little and appearing to get some relief from movement.

The thirst in *Rhus tox.* cases is as marked as it is in any drug in the materia medica; and the desire is for cold drinks. The restlessness of *Rhus tox.* is the main feature which distinguishes it from *Bryonia*, the other acute appendicitis drug. The appearance of the tongue is also a distinguishing feature between them. In practically all the acute complaints of *Rhus. tox.*, there is intense dryness of the tongue, and the appearance is always suggestive.

In typhoid and dysentery, the tongue tends to be red and scalded-looking all over. In acute appendicitis and acute gastritis, there is more likely to be a coating at the root of the tongue and a bright red, very sensitive, burning hot, dry tip.

In typhoid, the *Rhus tox.* patient tends to become very weak and develops a wandering, restless, very laborious type of delirium. In that state, the sleep is often very disturbed by nightmares of most violent physical exertion.

If the liver is involved and there is any jaundice, there is liable to be very intense skin irritation of the type one associates with the ordinary *Rhus tox.* eruptions.

SEPIA

THE typical *Sepia* digestive disturbance is a chronic, not an acute one, and the impression produced by the study of *Sepia* digestive disturbances is that the whole digestive mechanism is slowed down.

The patients suffer from a typical atonic dyspepsia. And they are liable to have a marked gastroptosis, even a marked visceroptosis, with a severe feeling of dragging and emptiness in the abdomen, which is not at all alleviated by eating.

Most *Sepia* patients one sees have had a long history of digestive difficulty. They give the story that they are always having sour, bitter eructations, their food does not seem to digest and, some hours after eating, the food is returned practically unchanged—except that it is sour and bitter.

They vomit all the food they have eaten and then, following the clearing of the stomach of the actual food material, they bring up a quantity of milky-looking fluid. This vomiting of milky fluid goes on indefinitely for hours after a meal.

With this atonic state of the digestion, the patients develop all sorts of desires for food with a definite taste—bitter, acid, vinegary, pungent—anything that has a bit of a kick about it. When the attacks are more acute, they develop an aversion to all food. In spite of the hungry, empty sensation, they do not want anything at all: the sight or, particularly, the smell, of food nauseates them.

In addition to their general drag and acidity, they get attacks of acute gastric pain. The peculiarity about the *Sepia* pain is that vomiting does not relieve it at all: it persists, or may even be aggravated, after they have vomited.

In addition to the gastric difficulty, there is the same atonic condition throughout the whole digestive tract. The patients suffer from what is popularly described as a sluggish liver. They are always conscious of a feeling of weight and drag in the region of the liver.

This dragging sensation is usually associated with a troublesome occipital headache. They are apt to suffer from very acute heartburn and burning, acid eructations which feel as if they scald the throat. There may be a degree of jaundice, and there is always very marked constipation.

In addition to the general liver disturbances, there is the same kind of torpid condition in the bowel. They suffer from intense flatulence, a feeling as if the whole abdominal contents were dragging down—and they appear to be just the type of patients that you would expect to get this disturbance.

They are typical visceroptotic, pot-bellied, flatulent, constipated people. Very often with these disturbances—either liver or flatulent constipation—you will find, on examination, large pigmented patches on the abdominal wall.

Associated with the bowel disturbances, there is commonly the most obstinate constipation. The pointer to the *Sepia* constipation is that after the bowels have acted, there is a feeling as of a great lump still left in the rectum which will not come away. The stools are always accompanied by the passage of a quantity of jelly-like mucus.

There will occasionally be a history of attacks of acute diarrhœa in *Sepia* cases, and again in the diarrhœa, the stool is always accompanied by a quantity of this jelly-like, whitish mucus, and after the bowels have acted there is a feeling as if there is a quantity of stool still to come away.

In addition to the general loathing of food, and nausea at the sight or smell of food, these *Sepia* patients very often have a marked aversion to milk and not infrequently are upset by it.

The impression I keep of the *Sepia* patient is one that might be expected as the result of the kind of physical make-up I have described: the tired-out, anæmic, depressed, miserable type of person, usually with a rather sallow complexion, very often with definite pigmented spots on the skin, very easily tired—mentally or physically—on any exertion, not wanting to do anything at all, wanting to be let alone and hating to be disturbed.

These patients always have a grievance: they have too much to do, or people are not kind to them, or no one realises how much suffering they have or with what difficulties they have to contend.

As one might expect in these tired-out patients with a grievance, they tend to be definitely bad-tempered, they resent criticism of any kind, are very liable to be spiteful and when things are too much for them, they are liable to burst into tears. Self-pity is one of the most outstanding characteristics of the *Sepia* make-up.

Sepia patients are always chilly, and sensitive to changes of temperature and electrical storms. They are very much better after a good long sleep; if they are wakened after a short sleep, they feel awful. Yet many of them say that they always wake in the mornings with an occipital headache, and feel more tired than when they went to bed and they very often feel sickish.

They are rather better after they get up and move about. Passive movement, however, such as riding in a car or train, is liable to make them feel worse, and may make them sick.

In women, all complaints—indigestion, constipation, liverishness, headaches, etc.—tend to be very much worse before and during the menstrual periods.

A peculiar thing about *Sepia* patients: in spite of their general tired, sluggish sort of state, they are peculiarly sensitive to noise. This usually produces the characteristic reaction of irritation and annoyance.

With vomiting of pregnancy, which is confined to the mornings and in which the patient has constipation, they may have slight headache on waking and vomit a quantity of whitish, milky-looking fluid, which will very often be controlled entirely by *Sepia*. This is particularly true if the patients have that strange *Sepia* empty hungriness most of the time and are very sensitive to the smell of cooking food.

SILICEA

OUR greatest use for *Silicea*, so far as digestive drugs are concerned, is probably in children; but sometimes there are indications for it in adults—in two different types of condition.

The first is the patient who has had a prolonged period of stress, is worn out nervously and suffering from nervous indigestion. This may show itself as a complete loss of appetite. Or it may take the form of a feeling of hunger on starting a meal, which is replaced by a sensation of extreme fullness after taking only a few mouthfuls of food.

Associated with a very definite aversion to anything in the way of hot food and hot drinks, a feeling as if the digestion just stopped, and a desire for everything cold—cold meat, ice-cream—such a condition very often responds, in these tired-out patients, to *Silicea*.

They mostly suffer from a good deal of flatulence, a feeling of general abdominal distension, a very acute feeling of fullness after meals (when their clothing feels too tight) and a certain amount of general abdominal tenderness.

They nearly always suffer from constipation and it is a great effort for them to get the bowels to act, straining at stool often makes them very hot and sweaty, and there is always a feeling as if the stool were partially expelled and then receded. They pass small constipated stools, and always feel that they have not nearly completed the action.

The other is the patient who has had a prolonged period of unsatisfactory physical conditions—bad feeding or unhealthy conditions generally—and who suffers from chronic diarrhœa.

These patients are in very much the same sort of tired-out state as those in the first group. Their diarrhœa is liable to be aggravated by milk. They are liable to suffer from very troublesome sick headaches, which are made much worse by any mental exertion and are aggravated by any noise. These are relieved by warm applications to the head, and also by pressure.

They are very much aggravated by any physical exertion, particularly stooping or the effort of talking. They usually start in the occipital region and spread right through the head, with the right eye as a centre. As a rule, they start some time after the patient gets up, usually during the forenoon; and they tend to get worse toward evening, as the patient tires.

Practically all these patients with chronic diarrhœa develop an acute aversion to meat. Most of them suffer from very troublesome sweaty feet.

Now for children. *Silicea* is one of the great standbys for those who suffer from a milk intolerance. This particularly in the child with a somewhat enlarged abdomen, probably some enlarged abdominal glands, a rather indefinite general abdominal tenderness and a history of alternate attacks of very obstinate constipation and very troublesome diarrhœa.

All these *Silicea* patients, whether old or young, are very chilly, but they are far more sensitive to damp cold than dry cold—in fact, most of them are better in a dry, fresh, cold atmosphere. They are all rather tired-out—nervously, physically, or both—and the condition produced is a very unpleasant feeling of inadequacy and a constant dread of making a mess of things. In actual fact, *Silicea* patients are really quite efficient.

The conditions which give rise to the *Silicea* state are very different from those which respond so well to *Nux*. *Nux* patients are fretted by dealing with a hundred and one irritations. *Silicea* patients, on the contrary, are tired out by a period of prolonged mental or physical stress which has worn them down.

Silicea patients tend to be rather timid, retiring and somewhat shy. When forced to do anything, or disturbed, they are apt to be irritable and snappish. In children, this is common: if they are left alone, they are quite peaceful; when disturbed, they are cross, and often cry and fight to get away.

Silicea patients with digestive disturbances tend to get exceedingly troublesome dry lips. The lips crack and very often develop deep, sensitive fissures at the angle of the mouth.

Most of these patients complain of cold, damp feet, very often with offensive perspiration. Under any stress, the head becomes extremely hot and perspires; if it gets chilled at this time, the result is liable to be a very acute headache. In summer, a similar headache is very likely to be produced by exposure to the sun. The head becomes very hot and extremely painful, and the pain persists for hours after exposure.